HOMEOPATHIC MEDICINE FOR MENTAL HEALTH

A homoeopathic doctor and psychiatrist shows how homoeopathy can be used to good effect in dealing with a wide range of emotional problems.

HOMEOPATHIC MEDICINE
FOR MENTAL HEALTH

A Self-Help Guide to Remedies that
can Restore Calm and Happiness ■

TREVOR SMITH, M.D.

HEALING ARTS PRESS
ROCHESTER, VERMONT

Healing Arts Press
One Park Street
Rochester, Vermont 05767

Note to the reader: This book is intended as an informational guide. The remedies, approaches, and techniques described herein are meant to supplement, and not to be a substitute for, professional medical care or treatment. They should not be used to treat a serious ailment without prior consultation with a qualified healthcare professional.

Printed and bound in the United States

10 9 8 7 6 5 4 3

Healing Arts Press is a division of Inner Traditions International

Distributed to the book trade in the United States by American International Distribution Corporation (AIDC)

Distributed to the book trade in Canada by Publishers Group West, Montreal West, Quebec

Distributed to the health food trade in Canada by Alive Books, Toronto and Vancouver

This book is dedicated with affection and gratitude to the memory of Dr Marjorie Blackie who so uniquely combined the qualities of homoeopath, teacher and healer.

CONTENTS

INTRODUCTION

The busy practitioner's surgery is never short of problems needing help and advice in a wide variety of ways. Some require a purely medical approach and prescription, others a surgical opinion, X-ray or specialized investigation. But, whatever the physical problem, every patient needs time, not only for examination and diagnosis, but, above all, time for support, reassurance and the all-important listening. However varied the complaints and difficulties, it is always the emotional ones which are most common and the present widespread social tensions, pressures and uncertainties are powerful factors in aggravating them. At least one patient in three now requests help for a problem which is directly psychological in origin and this is on the increase.

We are living in a society where there are demands for change and modification far beyond any expected norm of even ten years ago, and independent of the home environment - whether a country cottage or town flat. Especially, there are demands for an adjustment between the sexes, particularly from the newly 'liberated' woman, as differing roles, attitudes and reform bring increased opportunity and challenge. But, in order to be able to respond to and take full advantage of such opportunities, these changes must first be accepted psychologically, and not only at a functional level.

Deep personality adjustments always take longer to be accepted and integrated than those at a purely practical and organizational level, and during this age of psychological change, the woman is more vulnerable emotionally and more prone to illness and possible break-down. Less obviously, but equally profoundly, men are also involved in similar changes, although this is not always appreciated. They too have to rethink their traditional roles and attitudes, come to terms with a greater freedom of expression, opportunity and competition, accepting sharing in areas which, until recently, were solely masculine reserves.

With the threats of and realities of redundancy, not only the male, but the family as a whole has to be prepared to be a lot more flexible, able to accept new jobs and challenges in new areas. This may often mean work in quite different parts of the country, perhaps abroad. When open attitudes are present, the worker faced with redundancy, whatever his level, quite often finds that he has a surprising choice of challenging jobs available. For many years he may have been undervaluing his skills, underselling himself, closing his eyes to new and alternative growth prospects for the sake of security, and preserving the status quo. Only when faced with the reality of redundancy, do many realize that they have spent years in depressing, unrewarding employment, ignoring alternatives which offered expansion and opportunity.

To some extent, every couple is directly or indirectly affected by such changes, as the reassuring, old, familiar ways and patterns of traditional family life and morals are being questioned, challenged and found lacking. Because of present severe and widespread economic difficulties, redundancies, teenage unemployment and early retirement now threaten a very large percentage of the population, and almost every family is in some way directly involved in the resultant social anxiety and unrest. In one form or other, every community, however small, now has its share of social reaction — in the form of protests, sit-ins, or outbreaks of violence. It is not surprising that such manifestations and changes can also pose a threat and, in some cases, become a source of profound anxiety as they question established beliefs, individual life-styles, and values. Such pressures and disturbances can also precipitate a break-down, particularly where confidence and security are weakly established, so that the climate of political and social unrest seems unbearable, and heightens emotional problems and psychological tensions.

In times of war on the other hand, when there is a common, unifying, external enemy, healthy motivation is created, which allows negative hates and resentments to be harnessed and channelled positively, giving a raison d' être. When the enemy is less well defined, more of an internal one, involving the necessity for an adjustment of social attitudes within the individual and a pruning of government spending, then the drive and motivating forces are less or absent, and neurosis and break-down are common.

The over-anxious executive, threatened with failing business orders, worker-unrest and redundancy fears, is always under stress, which inevitably leads to irritability, heightened tension and nervousness. Feelings of defeat, depression, and insomnia are common. When the pressures are intolerable, there may be a complete nervous break-down.

The manual worker may express his worries more indirectly. Physical symptoms, perhaps frequent catarrh, colds, backache, raised blood pressure, indigestion or peptic ulcers are common. But there are no fixed patterns, and the underlying fears and anxieties may be expressed in a variety of ways.

Often it is the intimate relationship between husband and wife which bears the brunt of pressures. Impotence has now become increasingly common in a younger age group, with excessive evening fatigue after a busy, but essentially normal working day. There is just enough energy left to eat and watch television at the end of the day, but energy for nothing else. Problems of promiscuity, frigidity and marital breakdown, are also now very common, and flight from any real commitment to a relationship or family life is increasingly the rule rather than the exception.

With others, there is no direct psychological expression of underlying problems, either physically or emotionally, and they must emerge in other forms. It is increasingly common for many, of both sexes, especially the young adolescent and adult, to express their hostility and sense of defeat and resentment in more directly violent and anti-social ways. Feeling that the world owes them a living, that society should take care of them, they become increasingly dissatisfied, resentful, and irresponsible — anti-everything. There is denial of identification and responsibility, and a craving for the immediate. This usually means immediate sex, immediate money, immediate self-gratification, gambling, crime, and drugs, and this is evidenced by the spread of betting and sex shops. In older age groups, the same phenomena occurs, but the aggression occurs more indirectly, with widespread moral delinquency, so that, where possible, tax evasion and moonlighting have become increasingly the norm.'

A further factor in the development of psychological illness is the growing tendency towards passive and unimaginatively rigid attitudes. This is clearly seen in adult education classes and retraining centres, as much as in the schoolroom and the family. Indeed it is our educational system which is largely to blame, discouraging from the earliest years all form of originality, healthy questioning and spontaneity of thought in problem-solving in favour of a rigid examination system. This has led to a society which is largely rigid, repressed and uncreative in its attitudes to the resolution of present social problems. It has also unfortunately led to general indifference and a lack of awareness.

In society generally, there is a marked shortage of men or women of vision, imagination and leadership. Naturally such a fundamental lack of originality is also a danger to the individual and his flexibility in coping with seemingly insoluble adult problems. The young man with an ambition, an ideal, an aim, let alone a dream or a vision has become a rarity. Some of our most brilliant thinkers and leaders have undoubtedly been those who have escaped the system, through illness, or because they were considered to be such dunces as not to be worth bothering with. They were thus left to their own pathways and discoveries.

In any new learning situation, people now want to be told how to think, how to tackle a problem, or to know how someone else is going about it. They want to copy others, to be passively drilled, to learn by rote in parrot fashion. There is opposition to making the time to understand, develop the joy and the thrill of finding out, so discovering their own unique reactions and perceptions. This is the model — to identify rather than to discover and unfold within a learning situation.

There is another element and contributory factor to emotional illness closely related to the generalized passivity, which is quite simply that people don't really communicate any more, at least in any meaningful way. We have become a nation of watchers and spectators, addicted as much to the way we watch television, as on the sports field, rigid in the way we think and converse, and in our attitudes generally. Most of our leisure time activity, attitudes and behaviour are dominated and led by the media and, increasingly, we are in danger of becoming passive onlookers, rather than participants in any form of discussion and debate. Reading in some countries has become rare, and watching, listening, sitting back and resignation are the rule. This lack of conversation, through which opinions and feelings are shared, does little to foster understanding. An open, spontaneous dialogue and interchange of ideas is basic for any relationship to grow and remain strong and healthy, and is fundamental in the prevention of mental illness.

Causes of Emotional Illness
The causes of these disturbances are many and complex and include both environmental and hereditary factors; in particular, it is the quality of the earliest experiences and upbringing within the family which is the key to psychological health. The fulfilment of both physical and emotional needs are fundamental and basic to every child's growth of personality, confidence and intellect. However close the parents or comfortable the home, ultimately it is the consistent degree of warmth, attention, caring and loving appreciation shared openly within the family which is the basis for security. Such a background gives the best

protection against severe emotional pressures in later adult life, whatever the social and economic pressures at the time.

Naturally, all of us have 'scars' and even that idealized state of pre-natal, uterine bliss, can be far removed from an idyllic haven. Apart from the dangers of illness and infection during the early formative weeks, there are other more subtle problems for the growing foetus. These are shown by the fear reactions of the young foetus to any sudden jolting movements by the mother, or to loud external noises, as well as the less easily recorded stresses in response to toxins such as alcohol in excess, cigarette nicotine, environmental lead and drugs taken by or prescribed for the mother in pregnancy. Birth itself can often be a trauma, both psychologically as well as physically, particularly when it is at all precipitate or artificially induced, and damage or infection can occur before life has barely commenced.

For the majority, however, it is the earliest infantile experiences and disturbances, rather than the pre-natal or birth experiences which are the most significant in the cause and development of later neurosis and emotional disturbances. When the childhood experiences have been solid in the sense of recognition and acceptance as a person, where affection, physical contact and security is given quite spontaneously and freely without periods of sudden, undiscussed separation, then the adult is less likely to crumple into emotional illness and break-down when under pressure.

In some cases, individuals display an obsessional need to recreate earlier painful upsets and stresses in their contemporary adult world and relationships in a vain attempt to re-experience and master them. Although the unconscious aim of such an attempt may be to understand and to heal, too often infantile behaviour tends to be repetitive and intrinsically damaging, creating intolerable pressures. Usually this leads to a further sense of rejection and failure at the expense of the relationship, with few gains in understanding and caring for the individuals involved.

There are many trigger factors involved in emotional illness; some of these are purely physical in origin, especially in cases of debilitating and long, drawn out illnesses. In particular, influenza, glandular fever, shingles and hepatitis drain both the emotional and the physical reserves, often causing depression or emotional illness in one form or another. Alcoholism can be regarded as a debilitating addictive illness, damaging the body and mind, and can be a powerful contributing factor in a break-down. But frequently, the explanations given seem insufficient and there are no obvious precipitating pressures or stresses sufficient to cause illness. Often there has been a simple misunderstanding, or argument, the loss of a close friend or member of the family — a much-loved grandparent, important in earlier years. Any or all of these factors may lead to a sense of loss, insecurity and to feelings of rejection and abandonment.

In other cases, a colleague has been promoted, often a younger person; this is felt to be unfair, stimulating a sense of injustice and feelings of anger, resentment, or failure. Inevitably, there is a sense of judging the situation and of feeling unloved and unloving, unappreciated and undervalued. Also, there is sometimes a strong sense of being emotionally biased in one's appraisal of the situation, which does little, however, to stem the disturbing flood of hostility and resentment that bursts to the surface and leads to an added sense of failure and depression. Such emotional stirrings and reactions inevitably link up with infantile hurts at both a conscious and unconscious level. Often a double-hurt is experienced as the past is painfully relived through the apparent injustices of the present. It is these dual levels of emotion and pain which then act as a trigger to tip the balance into emotional break-down.

A mature adult relationship helps enormously to sustain a healthy emotional balance, preventing injured feelings and bruised reactions which can lead to severe loss of perspective, self-esteem and of confidence. The acceptance by the person of at least some responsibility for his illness is a further important and basic step in understanding and in softening rigid attitudes to make way for a more forgiving, caring outlook, which is an essential stepping stone to psychological health.

Homoeopathy and Emotional Illness

Since its origins over 150 years ago, homoeopathy has placed particular emphasis on the psychology of the individual. The concept of the person as a totality rather than as just a collection of inter-related anatomical parts has always played a fundamental role in the search for accurate diagnosis and positive treatment. As much attention is given to the individual's attitudes and the quality and depth of relationships formed as to the physical expressions of that person. The degree of stability, flexibility and involvement in society, and the ability to express as well as control feelings are all used in the homoeopathic profile.

The homoeopathic attitude to the patient with psychological problems is primarily one of a patient under intolerable emotional pressures. These may be expressed indirectly as a variety of physical disabilities which are not responding to treatment. Above all the patient is not seen as just another neurotic with a collection of irritating symptoms which he should learn to live with or take tranquillizers for. Homoeopathy makes no attempt to judge, criticize or moralize and is unique in its approach. Because the homoeopathic physician does not address himself to fragmented bits of the self which the patient desperately presents as his real being in a bid for help and attention, he is less distracted and sees the total picture more clearly. There is no emphasis on changing the person, his values or the way he sees the future. This area is left to the individual to work out for himself when stronger, and is a principle which reflects the fundamental trust in the ability of the healthy personality to resolve its own problems, hurts and distortions. Such strengths occur quite naturally through the action of the homoeopathic potencies, particularly when taken in the higher dilutions.

Because of the personal approach, the homoeopathic patient is not seen as a machine — in for servicing; homoeopathy is supportive as well as therapeutic. The concept of a patient coming for 'replacement of parts' is particularly inappropriate in any psychological condition, where the need is for consolidation and integration of existing strengths, feelings and emotions. This approach is, of course, more valid and appropriate when the patient is admitted to hospital for a transplant operation or valve replacement in a heart condition; but even when surgery is required, whenever the patient is acknowledged and treated as an intelligent person with genuine feelings, then the operation itself and convalescence period are smoother with less likelihood of complications developing.

When appropriate, the homoeopath uses all the conventional diagnostic investigations and procedures to clarify the cause of the disease. The homoeopathic doctor differs in some respects, however, from the practitioner of conventional allopathic medicine, which is based on concepts of treatment by opposites — with the emphasis on the suppression of symptoms. Using the conventional approach, when the patient is hot he is given a drug to cool him down, when excited, a substance to calm him down. By contrast, the homoeopath is opposed to all form of suppression of symptoms and of the individual. When the homoeopathic patient is hot and agitated he is given a remedy which, in its natural form, would provoke a similar feverish reaction — e.g. *Belladonna* or deadly nightshade. The same substance in its undiluted yet dynamic form, gives the homoeopath a tool to stimulate all the natural resources of the body and thus to lessen symptoms without putting the patient at risk. When there is depression, agitation or problems of anxiety, a remedy is chosen that if taken in its original unprepared state would provoke similar mental symptoms as a reaction to its toxicity — e.g. *Sepia*, the ink of the cuttle-fish.

In homoeopathy, synthetic drugs are not used, only natural source material which is toxic to man in its unprepared form, and therefore capable of evoking symptoms. Research studies called 'provings' have clearly demonstrated that such substances in their diluted remedy form have the power to stimulate health-giving 'similar' reactions in a normal healthy person. This ability of the remedies to produce similar symptoms is used by the homoeopath to act positively for the patient and is the reason why he talks of curing 'like by like'.

Basically, symptoms are important for many reasons, and are generally the normal, healthy reaction to pressure and stress — in fact, they are signs of vitality. When there is a state of severe exhaustion, particularly in the elderly, such a reaction may be lacking, so that a serious condition may be present without there being any marked signs of the disease — as with pneumonia. Such a state may also be artificially induced at any age by the prolonged taking of drugs such as steroids, which provoke a condition of symptom-inhibition, masking infection and thus permitting illness to establish a hold with minimal warning.

The homoeopathic prescription has the ability to liberate vital energies locked up in the body, so that a healthier self is experienced, with a greater sense of vitality, energy and well-being. In all cases, the homoeopath avoids suppression because this does not cure but simply pushes problems deeper under the mental skin of the patient and, at best, when there is a psychological problem, gives apparent or temporary relief whilst avoiding the essential problem and underlying anguish. This is also the reason why the homoeopath does not use tranquillizers or sedatives since they ultimately sedate the person and not just his problem. When such treatments have been given in the past, they tend to push the problem into a semi-dormant position, just beneath the surface, and frequently the problem is made worse, and at best is ineffective.

The homoeopath also avoids drugs of addiction since they create an added problem for the patient and because, ultimately, they undermine his faculties as a human being. In addition, all too often, they are dangerous, ineffective and simply add to the existing problems and anxieties, rather than helping to solve them. None of the homoeopathic remedies causes addiction, and the remedy may be stopped at any time without either physiological or psychological withdrawal occuring.

When psychological blockages occur, for whatever reason, emotional energy is not only repressed and pushed under, but it also attaches itself to certain key organs, for example the lungs, stomach or colon, and these are used as a new pathway for the expression of feelings. When under emotional pressure, certain patients react with an attack of asthma, heartburn, indigestion or colitis, depending upon which particular organ is 'sensitized' and used as an outlet. Such psychosomatic alternatives are not without their dangers, however, and it is always more healthy for the individual to express feelings directly, however strong, frightening and threatening they may be, rather than indirectly and vicariously through an organ that is not basically designed to convey such intense feelings.

Homoeopathy aims at a re-integration of the total self, with a lessening of unhealthy psychological regressions, blockages and isolation. The homoeopathic prescription and general approach towards the person helps lessen the denial of painful hurts and memories, which can then be more easily brought to the surface, recalled, understood and discussed. This quite naturally leads to a strengthening of personality, confidence and to greater insights. Being able to tolerate mixed feelings and painful memories, previously thought impossible, leads to a lessening of fragmentation and the related physical 'conversion' or psychosomatic symptoms, with a considerable release of energy, well-being and drive. With the correct remedy, there is a slow emergence of the bruised aspects of the personality into the light of more adult maturity and understanding, so that a softening of earlier resentments and scars can occur.

The advantage of homoeopathy is its inherent effectiveness and safety, and that it supports the natural energies of the individual. In the majority of conditions, the response to treatment compares favourably with conventional methods, and in many cases, particularly where there is an underlying emotional factor, the results are superior and far less unpleasant. In all cases, the treatment is free from the often disastrous side-effects of the typical allopathic prescription, and when the treatment is stopped, the patient does not slide back to his previous state of illness. Homoeopathic patients hold their gains, and are not dependent upon their pills once they have made an initial improvement.

It sometimes happens that after an initial improvement through homoeopathic treatment, an apparent set-back occurs when nothing seems to be happening. This is quite usual and reflects a period of consolidation of response, while the body's defensive healing energies are being mobilized. Such a delay requires a degree of patience from the patient and his family, and it may cause problems when tension and impatience is marked, or where there is a long-standing problem with all the inevitable uncertainties and fears as to diagnosis, response to treatment and outcome. When there is a chronic problem, responses are inevitably slower, since the body takes time to recover from the underlying condition, depleted energy reserves, and often from the effects of previous treatments.

When an emotional problem has been suppressed over the years and the usual drugs are suddenly reduced or stopped, there is frequently a 'Jack-in-the-box' effect as the problem seems to recur with a vengeance. This may also occur at the start of homoeopathic treatment, and may cause a lot of anxiety. Usually such a 'blow out' is short-lived, and at times is mistakenly attributed to the homoeopathic remedies, rather than viewed as an inevitable consequence of long-term suppressant measures. In most cases, after a few days, the apparent worsening of symptoms quietens down, and a true improvement begins. In some cases, such a violent reaction may undermine the confidence of the patient, and cause a flight from homoeopathy back to more radical suppressants, perhaps even a return to stronger drugs than before. The priority for such patients is always immediate symptom relief, rather than ultimate cure, whatever the cost to the person himself and his underlying personality development.

During the course of the treatment, there may be a return of physical or mental symptoms not seen for years and which were not dealt with adequately at the time. These may be earlier problems, attitudes or fears, but usually such responses are intuitively understood by the patient as part of cure, because the general well-being is not lessened. Such responses are always an encouraging sign indicating a strong positive reaction to treatment, as the remedy works to loosen up remnants of illness. When such symptoms come to the surface they can be considered in terms of making way for a more free self, giving an increased depth of understanding and meaning in areas previously blocked and distorted and therefore incomprehensible. All of this broadens the picture and deepens understanding for both doctor and patient, and is an important part of the homoeopathic caring and cure. As subsequent layers emerge and old symptoms and attitudes are looked at, the totality of the individual can be treated with the most fitting remedy . In general, the aggravation is short-lived, quickly giving way to a period of more definite improvement.

Many conventional treatments deplete both body and mind, particularly the antibiotics, psychotropic drugs and tranquillizer group. All too often, they provoke reactions of lethargy, fatigue and exhaustion, worsening the underlying problem, or themselves creating symptoms through their side effects, which often resemble the original psychological problem. A very common symptom of emotional illness is this problem of exhaustion, and by conserving the essential energies, homoeopathy has the advantage of not provoking reactions of artificial lethargy and fatigue.

Because of ignorance and myth, there is still a lot of confusion about homoeopathy — what it is and how it acts — on the part of the general public and also the medical profession. It is often wrongly confused with herbalism, because some of the remedies originate from plant extracts. But many are also of animal and mineral origin, or prepared from tissues like vaccines, but without the usual dangers and side effects. These have an important role to play in the prevention and treatment of various specific infections, which may lead to severe states of chronic fatigue and depression.

Homoeopathy is not suggestion, nor is it a system of cure-all patent medicines. It is a complete and total scientific system of treatment, respected, accepted and taught throughout the world. In the U.K., it is prescribable on a health service prescription. Increasingly, more and more people turn to homoeopathy as a first-line treatment and approach to illness, rather than just an alternative to failed conventional methods.

The question often arises as to whether a patient should change his doctor for a homoeopathic one. Provided that the conventional treatment is satisfactory and there is a good, sensitive, understanding and open relationship where doubts and queries can be expressed, there is often no reason to change. When powerful drugs have been prescribed for an excessive period, often months rather than weeks, in some cases for years, this can obviously be both undesirable and potentially dangerous. In some cases, such prolonged treatments are a necessity, but for many they are not justified. In all cases, it should be possible to openly discuss the prescriptions given and the period of treatment with the doctor who prescribes. However, there is a growing number of thinking people who object to polypharmacy or multiple-drug prescribing, often on a repeat-prescription basis. They object to the excessive and routine prescribing of sedatives, tranquillisers, steroids and anti-depressants, often from an early age and are very concerned to avoid the dangers, albeit frequently unknown, of long-term prescribing and drug-induced illness. For such people homoeopathy offers a viable alternative, particularly in the area of emotional illness. But no treatment, whatever the condition or diagnosis, should be stopped abruptly without first consulting a physician, particularly where drugs have been prescribed over a period of several weeks.

For the majority, homoeopathic remedies act deeply and the results are positive. Where the main problem is of an emotional or mental nature, then in most cases my experience has clearly shown that it is the higher potencies or greater dilutions of 30c and above, up to the 200c, which give the best results at depth within the personality. Particularly the constitutional or 'overall' prescription which fits the general physiological and psychological make-up, trends of energy, metabolic activity and psychological attitudes has been proved time and time again to be of enormous value at various stages in life and often at times of crisis. It is nearly always prescribed in highest potency or maximum dilution of at least 200c and often the 10M dilution is used by many practitioners with good result. This constitutional remedy is frequently needed at various times throughout life and has the ability to unlock rigid or distorted patterns of perception and therefore of judgement.

A feeling of calm, happiness and well-being is usually achieved and because of its deep action in the mental sphere, emotional problems, previously thought insoluble, can be looked at in a more positive relaxed way. This leads to a more easy acceptance of an imperfect world and helps to lessen the distortion experienced by the patients. The growth achieved by such recognitions, facilitated by the remedy, leads to greater awareness and the resolution of underlying attitudes and problems can finally begin, allowing the subsequent development of greater self-confidence and maturity.

1.

THE ROLE OF THE HOMOEOPATHIC DOCTOR IN EMOTIONAL ILLNESS

We are living in a social climate of division and nowhere is this more evident than in our health service. It would be more accurate, in many ways, to say 'illness service' because, certainly, the emphasis does not seem to be on health and its preservation. Lip service only is paid to such fundamentals as the underlying causes of disease and its prevention, especially where psychological health is concerned. In general the service is bureaucratic, unimaginative and impersonal, primarily concerned with the treatment of symptoms of disease, rather than with people or the underlying psychological influences of all illness. Psychological problems in particular are largely neglected and the psychiatric patient is treated as a symptom or problem carrier, rather than as an individual that needs consistent support and understanding. On the whole the major preoccupation of the health service is one of investigation and treatment at the cost of personal caring and attention.

All too often the doctor himself is a victim of the many social pressures and divisions which beset us, becoming either a technician or an administrator. Nowhere is this more marked than in the field of emotional problems where too often, through shortage of time or inadequate training, he is under pressure and unable to understand the patient's needs in any depth. The doctor is in danger of becoming completely isolated and alienated from the true art of medicine, from healing and man's relationship to his essential inner self, his nature, faith, and the spiritual needs of each of us.

All too often, the modern patient is increasingly preoccupied and over-conversant with the external manifestations of his problems and with the names and colours of the tablets he is presently taking. However, he is isolated from his unconscious, from intuitiveness and from the deeper meaning and cause of his malaise. In the consulting room he is often confused, putting the wrong emphasis on the wrong feelings, asking the wrong questions, or worse — none at all. Acting in an artificial way, he adds further to his own confusions and those of the doctor, because of the uncertainty with which he presents himself and communicates. He has lost his essential simplicity and naivety.

All of this leads inevitably to faulty understanding in the surgery or out-patient department, with a false, distorted doctor-patient relationship, the wrong diagnosis and wrong treatment. There is no longer a depth and rapport in the relationship which could form the basis of a pathway to the development of insights, with a better understanding of the illness and its causes.

All too often, the G.P. sees his role as that of a referring agent rather than as a physician in any Hippocratic sense of the word — and so too does the patient. The doctor has become a kind of bureau, an office, where the patient collects certificates and prescriptions and is referred to the specialist. 'Specialist' in the patient's mind, and often in the doctor's, is equated with the *élite*, and 'the best for the patient'. But is it the best? The general physician, as he was formerly, hardly exists any more. All too often within the group practice, as it is now practised, the patient barely knows who is his doctor. He has become a number in a computer or filing system. Often he sees a different doctor in the surgery, according to his problems or the doctors' rota. At weekends he may see a doctor on call from an entirely different group practice, who knows nothing about the patient or his problems. The doctor in such a situation has probably never seen the patient before, and will probably never see him again.

For the majority of doctors, referral to the specialist or to hospital for a second opinion and investigation is both taught and believed to be the essence of good medical practice. The doctor must know his limitations and often feels he is not doing the best for the patient if he does not pass on the problem or call for a second opinion. In some countries, where litigation is a way of life, pressures to refer and to hand over the patient are even stronger because the doctor needs to protect himself whenever there is the slightest doubt as to diagnosis and the outcome of treatment. In some cases the pressures are so great that doctors have given up medical practice altogether, largely due to the high cost of malpractice insurance.

A patient was recently in hospital for the refitting of a cardiac pacemaker. The patient also had gall-stones. She mentioned this to her surgeon, who said that he was a 'heart doctor', and that he knew nothing about abdominal problems, but he would ask another surgeon to see her from another department — gastro-enterology — and advise. Presumably the other doctor knew nothing about heart problems. The patient, naively perhaps, only wanted to know whether the gall-stones could be dealt with at the same time as the fitting of the pace-maker and under the same anaesthetic. All she wanted was information — not a division of caring.

All such divisions make for severe fragmentation of the health service, playing havoc with the possibility of a good doctor-patient relationship developing. In the majority of cases within the hospital system, there is no pretence of any continuity of caring and, whether in the out-patient department or as an in-patient, patient responsibility is divided. The division exists to a varying degree between the consultant, registrar, houseman, medical student and the inevitable locum. The same is largely true of nursing care, where there are divisions between the regular trained day-staff, pupil nurses, nursing tutors and a variety of night staff coverage, including agency nurses, who vary from night to night and know least of all about the patient.

The exception only exists in the private sector where, in most cases, the patient sees the same doctor regularly and consistently, from admission until discharge. The patient is usually well informed and is generally treated as an intelligent human being and thinking person. In general the nursing care is also far more consistent and where agency nurses are used, these are often hired on a regular, long-term basis, which makes for greater nurse-patient continuity during the treatment. The non-private patient is lucky if he sees the consultant more than once on admission and even that does not always occur. It is quite common for there to be no discussion or explanation after the operation or treatment and all too often the patient is left completely in the dark as to the exact findings and what was done in a surgical procedure.

Apart from the private sector, there is only one other exception to such appalling confusion and fragmentation of treatment and that is in the increasingly rare cottage hospital system. In the few that now exist, there is still some continuity; the G.P. sees the patient throughout the treatment, may assist at an operation if necessary, and is there and available as a recognizable caring figure. There is a complete and ideal system of caring, also incorporating after-care. But this is rare and many of the old cottage hospitals, staffed by the local G.P.s and nurses, have closed down from lack of funds and support.

The argument in favour of a system of referral and of specialized medicine is a weak one. It is based on the assumption that with increasing knowledge, progress and sophistication, no physician could possibly keep abreast of so much new information. However, if one looks back at the field of mental problems which concern us, over the past twenty years, one finds that, in fact, there have been no significant advances in either diagnosis or treatment. The same drugs are still being prescribed as before — sometimes with some minor modification of formula or presentation, but essentially the same. Not uncommonly, some of the patients have been on those same drugs for most of the two decades. However much progress may have been made in the field of surgery and investigation techniques generally, as far as mental illness is concerned, there have been no major insights or changes which have emerged. Certainly in the handling of patients, there are fewer locked wards, but basic treatments and attitudes have changed little, and the frequency of anxiety, phobic illness and depression is, if anything, on the increase and is certainly no less frequent than in the 1960s.

If we now consider the different types of treatment generally available for emotional problems, we find that they fall into two distinct camps — the dynamic or psychotherapeutic/analytic approach and the more conventional/drug-based physical approach, which is based on and orientated towards behaviour modification. The doctor has the problem of initially sorting out which approach is best for a particular individual. Usually this is quite an impossible task, since the doctor lacks both the skill, time and training to be able to judge and differentiate between the two approaches. The treatment of psychological illness is one of the most neglected areas of medical training. Usually the G.P. must fall back on the local psychiatric unit or mental hospital, or often a specialist he has known in his training days or medical school. In many ways the latter choice is often preferable because at least there is usually a relationship between G.P. and consultant, which makes for the possibility of a dialogue developing concerning the patient, the management of his case and the likely outcome of his illness, all of which are of key concern to the patient and his family.

Both approaches inevitably have their limitations. In general, the dynamic school tends to be too remote, drawn out, theoretical and intellectual, despite the basic concern for the feelings of the individual. The dynamic therapist is interested in concepts and ideas — the influence of early infantile phantasy on present relationships. This is of value and tremendously important, but the therapist is usually forbidden to touch or examine the patient and any spontaneity of approach must be carefully controlled. The basic analytic approach allows for the emergence and significance of unconscious phantasy material, parental relationships and regression as relevant to the patient's treatment.

Psychotherapy, which is analysis in a less intense form, has the same drawbacks of the analytic approach. The common criticism is that treatment is too slow, not generally available for the majority of patients and not suitable because of the treatment fees which mount up over a prolonged period. In other cases, the type of problem, personality, background or age of the person, makes it unsuitable as a valid treatment. Where there is a need for basic development of personality and the patient cannot use his natural environment, then the foundation provided by the analytic or psychotherapeutic type of relationship is invaluable. Growth may occur which would be impossible in any other situation. Many, however, criticize the dynamic approach for being too contrived, and argue that all too often the criteria for acceptance into such treatment are so narrowly defined that they exclude the majority.

As described earlier, in order to keep the therapy 'pure', all physical contact with the patient is taboo. Traditionally, the analytic type of treatment is very concerned not to gratify any of the patient's unconscious wishes — particularly if they involve physical contact or stimulation in any way — in order not to arouse additional phantasies in this area. Because of this approach to the physical, when the patient is 'really' ill, he must then be referred to another doctor — his 'physical' doctor. Once again, there is a division of therapy, of communication and of the relationship. This makes for a division of the person too. He is told in analytic or dynamic therapy: 'Here we only deal with the psyche — not the body, not the whole person', in much the same way as the cardiac patient who was told: 'Here we only deal with the heart — not the abdomen.'

There are other dynamic therapies, in which the aim is more to do with manipulating the patient. Such therapy groups are usually given various primitive-sounding names, and tend to encourage a contrived, unhealthy regression technique, involving acting out within the group one's deepest needs and fears. This can be a very unwise exercise for certain types of personality, particularly the vulnerable or imaginative. Such an artificial catharsis is very rarely of any lasting therapeutic value, whatever the personality, and is rarely in the patient's real interest. Many of the regressive phenomena are of a contrived, hysterical nature and the patient gains nothing by exposing himself to unnecessary risks, particularly when he is in any way vulnerable or displays latent schizoid tendencies. The expense to the patient and family in both time, energy and monetary terms is often considerable.

The principles and techniques of modern conventional psychiatry are always to suppress or to change and modify, as opposed to the release of weakly integrated parts of the self, and their realignment into a position of growth of personality. Self-realization and insights into the personality are usually non-existent. In general, powerful and potentially dangerous drugs are used, often experimentally, to try to break down existing and established patterns of behaviour; sedatives, tranquillizers or anti-depressants are prescribed in varying degrees of high dosages. In the past, other equally radical and ineffective techniques have been used, including LSD and deep insulin coma treatment. In general, this approach treats the person as if he were just a bundle of neurological reflexes or an experimental animal rather than a dignified human being. Also, such eradicated symptoms must inevitably reappear, in a new, sometimes more dangerous form than in the original illness. A masochistic approach can never lead to any new learning or new growth by the patient, however humanely it is applied. With few exceptions, the physical and mechanistic approach pays little attention to the underlying feelings of the person or to the unconscious motivations which play a role in all emotional illness. Problems such as pride, jealousy, competition, loss or old resentments and scores are, for the most part, dismissed either as irrelevant, or as figments of the mind. The mechanistic approach is unimaginative because it makes no allowance for unconscious motivations; it makes for a purely mechanistic patient and this can be quite clearly seen after treatment when, all too often, the patient emerges more like an automatum doll than a person. For many, the neurotic position, with all its pains and tortuous tensions, is infinitely preferable to a drug-based masochistic 'cure'.

Medicine and the art of healing, as practised by Hahnemann and his colleagues, was a far cry from the medicine of today — it did not just involve the writing of a prescription or a form for specialized investigation. Essentially it was a therapy, although never called as much. Indeed, the very word had not been invented then; there was no need either since therapy was still an integral part of medicine. In those days, there was no need for therapy as such because the doctor practised a total and complete form of medicine and encompassed the roles of doctor, therapist and psychiatrist.

All of this quite naturally gave strength and confidence to the patient. It is also true that Hahnemann lived at a time before there was severe fragmentation of the family patterns, and could therefore more easily involve the whole family in a discussion, should it be in the patient's best interest. Such traditional approach is now called family therapy. The early physician also had the advantage of knowing the family as a whole — sometimes over several generations — which gave insights into habits and attitudes in a more general way. But above all, it was the doctor's open attitude that was the key to his success in treatment.

The homoeopath today also looks at all aspects of his patient — his family, background, physical and mental health — nothing is taken for granted before coming to a decision on treatment. Again, like the early physicians, the homoeopath takes the blood pressure, examines the bowels, abdomen or skin — whatever is necessary to reassure the patient and complete the examination and diagnosis. He also listens to the patients dreams and fears. Less rarely is there a referral for a second opinion. It is certainly no routine and, when necessary, it is fundamental that there is a communication between the referring doctor and the specialist with no loss of the patient to a system. Should surgery be required, the homoeopathic remedy and approach, both before and after the operation supports healing, directing the body and mind to smooth the recovery.

The homoeopath is not a specialist, other than in the toxic-pictures of the remedies he uses. He is closer to the early physicians, indeed a continuation of them, taking a much more central position than either the drug-oriented psychiatrist or the dynamic analyst or psychotherapist when dealing with emotional problems. His aim is always to support the healthy aspects of personality and to avoid unnecessary infantile or regressive behaviour or flight into illness. He does not suppress or judge whatever the patient expresses, but examines it, shares an interest and is attentive to all aspects of the individual's make-up. Physical symptoms such as cramps at night, psoriasis or varicose veins, are just as important and as relevant to the homoeopath as childhood patterns of upbringing, sibling rivalry and old resentments, and physical problems often contribute to emotional difficulties. Being less rigid, not tied to dogma or unbending patterns and prescriptions, the homoeopath naturally helps the patient to be less anxious and dogmatic, more easy and spontaneous. Above all, he is ordinary in his approach, not grand or special; he works with the patient on an equal basis in a sort of partnership, thereby encouraging patients to be more open and natural and above all to be themselves.

Homoeopathy places particular emphasis on the factors which aggravate or improve the underlying problem. Any group of unusual symptoms — the 'odd, rare and peculiar' can also give the clue to diagnosis and accurate prescribing. All of this is explained to the patient — the homoeopath does not play God.

Homoeopathic remedies avoid side effects or 'doctor-induced' illness. Problems such as muscular rigidity, drowsiness, malaise, fainting, weakness, nausea, Parkinsonism and jaundice do not occur as complications of homoeopathic treatments. A remedy is not given if it is a danger to the patient, nor is a treatment prescribed that will make the patient worse by creating an artificial symptom or illness. The remedy has only one function — to stimulate the natural healing resou ces present in every individual, and to support and strengthen all aspects of him as a human being. The fundamental aim is to balance the person psychologically whenever judgement and perspective are out of true. Particularly the remedies prescribed in their highest potencies act at this level, and often quickly. The homoeopath aims to enable the patient to act more positively and logically, and to be able to come to decisions about the quality of his life and goals, often avoided over many years as new and frightening or too much of a challenge.

It is quite a frequent occurrence to see a patient who becomes impotent as a result of his drug treatment — the tablets he is taking for blood pressure or depression. Too often such impotence is accepted as inescapable and a natural consequence of treatment, without questioning why the individual is really ill and the reasons for it in terms of his attitudes and lifestyle. The passivity of many patients and the lack of questioning with regard to the drugs they are taking and their implications is frightening.

Having a healthy attitude towards his patients, the homoeopath aims to stimulate the healthy aspects of the patient and his personality. The remedies encourage a release of earlier resentments or old attitudes, of punishment, rage and unforgiveness, which all too often rise to the surface, causing emotional problems and symptoms. Such unhealthy attitudes are often long-standing and directed at the parents and family. Often, mental illness is nothing more than a continuation of such distorted immature infantile attitudes, directed at others who happen to be in the individual's pathway or environment at the time.

The homoeopath makes no demands of his patient other than to take the prescribed remedies regularly and to avoid damaging his body and mind with a diet which is excessive or dangerous. The remedy is always based on individualization, and is the one which best fits the particular attitudes, difficulties and symptoms of the time. The doctor then waits to see the effects of the remedy upon the total system and the changes in the patient.

If there is a call for the physician to be more of a person and a man, and less of a bureaucrat, administrator and technician, in the tradition of the great men of medicine — Osler and Hippocrates — so too does the patient need to be more of a person, taking far more responsibility, not only for his sickness, but also for how it is treated, and ultimately how he himself is cared for. This is linked with the degree that the patient ultimately cares for himself and for others. The patient also needs to be more of a thinker, more willing to examine his feelings and to work at greater understanding of and insight into self and the reasons for illness.

Viewing illness as an unfortunate happening, a collection of external circumstances, nothing at all to do with the patient, all too often avoids his own role and contribution to his sickness and is not helpful. The patient must learn to be less of an automaton, less of a pillbox, and not just an empty container for other people's ideas, opinions and medicines. All too often the patient becomes sluggish and is depersonalized by his various pills over the years and then wonders why the results are so unsatisfactory.

Much greater responsibility is needed then by both patient and doctor. The patient must learn to appreciate how he can harm himself and contribute to his illness through unhealthy attitudes and denial. He further contributes to his own condition through excessive eating and smoking. Excessive weight and dietary excess needs to be curbed and thought more about before it becomes a danger to health, sometimes to life. Regular exercise and healthy stimulation of the body and mind are essential for all of us, and increased awareness should be an important part of daily caring and meditation. Similarly, the amount of alcohol and tobacco consumed should be kept to sensible proportions, and if this is not possible, it should be discontinued totally. With the patient playing a more active part in the prevention of his illness, thinking more about the needs of the body and mind, there will follow a natural progression away from passivity, away from suppression and suppressant treatments as the self becomes more highly valued — opening the way to a more healthy world generally.

2.

EMOTIONAL PROBLEMS OF
THE INFANT

During these early years, the character and personality is built up and established so that any emotional problems that occur are centered around this essential process — primarily one of growth and natural maturation. Character and personality develop by a complex series of perceptions, explorations and contacts with the outer world and especially with the people in it. There is a need for each infant to find out for himself his own position in this world and to identify his degree of acceptance with those who have grown up in it. Having tested out the realities of the external world and ascertained its boundaries, the infant is more able to move out into the world, express himself within it and develop his own points of view on it. There is a constant review of these experiences of reality and how the individual relates to them, revising the limitations of behaviour as well as that which is permitted and tolerated. Confidence and experience is built up, layer by layer, with each new acquisition of vital experience, reflecting a growth of knowledge as each satisfactory experience and contact builds up a depth reflecting the uniqueness of the individual.

Of course the relationship with parents, grandparents and siblings are all part of the key to stability, self-reliance and trust in the self that is formed and extended. The earliest explorative steps into self-confidence are often by means of games, play and fairy stories. In the older child, similar explorations are continued in multiple relationships with people at school, including teachers and other children — both in learning and in sports. Each new experience and relationship adds a dimension, a building up of earlier experiences. Whenever there is a healthy physical growth it is accompanied by a parallel emotional one. Similarly, emotional growth is accompanied by healthy physical development. These processes occur quite naturally with little encouragement, since each step or experience is one of growth and confidence.

Heredity plays a role in these developments, as can be clearly seen by observing the temperamental differences between twins — even identical ones. This difference is often very considerable and is not accounted for by any difference in environment or parental attitudes.

But by far the most important factor in the healthy integration and building up of security and personality lies within the family — its degree of stability, flexibility, understanding and love which is provided and shown. The degree of closeness and affection, given both overtly and in more subtle ways, is the key to the development of a child's confidence as well as his ability to display similar feelings throughout life. The fullest development of affection and caring is further encouraged by unrestricted physical holding of closeness with the child during infancy and throughout childhood.

A secure relationship with the mother is always vital, whatever the sex, the culture or family patterns. But a sound relationship with both parents is also important for security to be fully established. Such a relationship implies that there is a good sharing between the parents, excluding the possibility of a very disturbed child using manipulation or unwarranted, emotional outbursts to split off one of the parents or to reject them. The parents need at all times to maintain a balanced, central position which does not allow for such manipulations or the excessive interplay of sibling jealousies and the inevitable rivalries that occur in every family — usually based on fear and insecurity.

When there is a one-parent family, the position is rather different; although the same problems occur, they are often expressed through other adult figures, and security is sometimes indirectly worked out via other members of the family or community as are available and involved with that family. These are quite clearly seen by the growing child as parent-substitute figures and all their feelings are naturally tested out on them in an endeavour to stimulate natural feedback-responses for their essential learning, developing and growth. In general, when there is a sense of openness, security and relaxation between the parents or parent-substitutes this makes for security in both children and the adults concerned. It is imperative that the need of feedback and response is understood and not just seen as childish demands which are senseless and irritating.

These attitudes and relationships between the parents are far more important than any material considerations for the developing child's security and future strengths. Such attitudes are accurately perceived and sensed by the healthy child as an integral part of the images he uses to build up a picture of the adult world — primarily of the parents, but also of adult life in general. When the images are solid with a degree of genuine togetherness, sharing, support and loving, such feelings are built into the child's perceptions of its world and life, becoming a part of his roots and deepest self.

A child will quite naturally develop strengths of personality and confidence, with a feeling of developing self-reliance, provided that this has not in any way been impeded by the parents or by any of their individual problems. In a community or kibbutz type of upbringing, the parents are still psychologically essential as part of the child's secure model for the future — to identify with and to rely upon, whatever the hereditary endowment. Whenever security is disturbed because these parental models are absent or interfered with in any way, then the psychological growth of the child may be severely affected.

Unfortunately, interference and interruption of such natural processes can occur at any time, affecting the sensitivity, natural flexibility and resilience of the individual child. Such psychological pressures usually come from within the family, sometimes from physical trauma or illness, and all too often such pressures result in break-down at sometime.

Any form of separation from or death of a parent or sibling can be critical in these formative years. Rejection by a parent, even a physical assault or baby battering during a period of depression or alcoholism is not uncommon. A further trauma is more subtle and the result of repeated and constant physical upheaval and changes of home and school which, if repeated, are undermining to the healthiest child — the constant uprooting of friendships, home, environment and culture is disturbing to the developing child as well as to his parents. In such a situation the parents may reflect their own anxiety by their handling of the increasingly demanding and anxious child. All of this interferes with the very roots and security of personality and physical growth and is often a cause of the profoundest depression.

When the earliest experiences have been unduly negative, leading to a kernel of bitter experiences, this can be almost like a 'growth' taking on a life of its own and leading to a sense of permanent dissatisfaction and rejection, of being unloved, that seems impossible to resolve however sensitive and caring relationships become at a later date.

Infantile and Child Anxiety States
This condition is commonly seen when the background is insecure and when there is uncertainty within the family — perhaps the parents are unsure of themselves and just how to relate to or handle the child's many complex demands and needs. When this happens, the easiest solution for many adults is simply to try and stifle the child selfishly for the sake of peace and quiet. For some children there may have been an

acute trauma — the sudden loss of a parent, brother or sister from illness, the family overwhelmed and quite unprepared for such a loss. In others there has been a tragic sudden suicide in the family — perhaps a close relative and ripples of guilty feelings felt in every member of the family and somehow allowed to concentrate in the child. Sometimes one of the parents is being treated for severe depression, or there is chronic tension between the mother and father, or problems of compulsive drinking or gambling, the resulting anxiety and tensions reflected in their handling of the child and not just emerging as tensions between the adults.

When the background is at all uncertain or unloving in any way, this is naturally sensed by most children, with increased needs for reassurance and attention. Feelings of guilt are common in adults and at times these may be projected into a young and vulnerable child, highlighting confusion and anxiety. Not uncommonly, the child has been prematurely exposed to some form of adult sexuality, molested or interfered with in some way, even the victim of an actual rape or physical assault. Such damage in some cases is provoked by the immature child turning inappropriately to a stranger for affection when the home environment is lacking in understanding or where there are severe clashes and problems within the parental relationship.

With others, the damage is more subtle and difficult, with adult feelings and problems thrust upon the child's shoulders before he is mature enough to understand and contain them. This particularly may be a problem in certain one-parent families or when there is alienation within a marriage, the underlying emotional problems not discussed or worked through by the parents. Not uncommonly there is also a familial or hereditary disposition towards nervousness and emotional problems which is passed to the sensitive child with added complications of nervousness and tension.

The problems of the nervous and sensitive child do not occur in isolation and when there are underlying problems between the parents, these may come to the surface when the child becomes more 'difficult', demanding or unwell. The mixture of anxiety, fear and guilt often increases pressure on the parents, even increasing arguments, fatigue, tension and recrimination, rather than bringing them together.

The major symptoms of childhood anxiety are basically those of fear and restlessness; fear of leaving home, eating lunch at school, the need to run home to see that everything is 'alright'. Sometimes this centres around fears of something happening to one of the parents, particularly the mother or a sibling, when the child is at school. This may also lead to problems of truancy, fabricating stories, at times to pilfering or, more worrying, to stealing from outside the immediate family. Others behave in a more serious, attention-seeking way, bordering on delinquency, by starting fires in the classroom, playing with matches or any dangerous game so that they become a threat to buildings or crops and to others.

There may be many physical symptoms of a child's anxiety, particularly problems such as bed-wetting, being faddy with foods, clumsiness, tearfulness, or odd abdominal pains which do not fit into any recognizable medical diagnosis. Eczema, asthma, and increasing proneness to infection of the throat and catarrhal problems are all common manifestations of the disturbed child, particularly when there is a family and constitutional tendency to weakness in these areas. Increased accident-proneness can be another manifestation of the disturbed child — somehow always in a wrong position and off-balance, whatever the situation.

When the parents are naturally sensitive and intuitive, able to share and discuss these needs and problems with the child, then their frequency and severity are greatly reduced and may more often be contained. When both parents are out at work, and the mother is not home when the child returns from school in the afternoon, then such problems that arise are more difficult to understand and deal with because they are not seen as they occur, and the mother, indeed both parents, may be exhausted by their own problems, their job and the travelling. Given such circumstances, the problems that arise in any family may be increased with an added tendency to babyish demanding ways. However good the grandparents are at such times, when there is a real crisis they can, at best, usually only contain it temporarily; there are no real substitutes for the listening ear or enveloping arm of the child's actual parents.

The Commonest Emotional Problems, Their Symptoms and Some Homoeopathic Remedies

Insecurity and Fear

The child is agitated and unable to settle and play in any constructive or involved way. These children always seem to be restless, preoccupied and in need of constant help and attention, demanding to be held or have an adult within close proximity. Sleep is a common problem, the child waking frequently with disturbed dreams from fear, exhausting the parents. Often the child eventually ends up sleeping in the parents' bedroom so that they can obtain some essential rest. When the child is irritable and sleeping badly because of teething problems *Chamomilla* is of value, especially when the child cries as soon as put down to rest and if not held constantly. The exact remedy varies with the particular child and his temperament, but remedies to be considered include *Valerium,* *Calcarea, Lycopodium, Gelsemium* and *Passiflora.*

The Over-active Child

This is a common problem and an exhausting one. The child is excessively anxious, often psychologically damaged and deprived, constantly on-the-go and clinging to any adult figure in the vicinity, often in an exaggerated, over-affectionate manner. The other common cause is a traumatic one following a precipitate delivery requiring either forceps or a last-minute repositioning of the foetus. The child comes through the birth canal much too quickly for the head to adapt to the pressures and there is a degree of damage to the nervous system. Such damage, although sub-clinical in the sense of not sufficiently severe to provoke a recognizable clinical illness, does damage the child and provoke disturbances of temperament with an inability to relax. Often such a child cannot be easily controlled without an adult constantly being in the vicinity to see that it does not damage either itself or an article of furniture in its fidgeting searches. In addition, they are often very well developed children, and physically very strong.

The remedy that is most useful is *Arnica,* followed by *Helleborus* and *Veratrum alb.* when there is a history of precipitate birth shock and damage. Such children are also very bright and an early entry to nursery school is recommended. The child's constitutional remedy should be given in high potency at an early stage and repeated frequently. Often response and improvement is slow when the over-activity and underlying anxieties take origin from within the family following a period of loss or separation with isolation and fear; these difficulties need to be carefully understood and discussed with the child at the appropriate moment in order to reassure fears and to explain what may be a terrifying experience with the overwhelming fear of a repetition.

School Phobias

In many cases there is an emotionally depressed, sometimes phobic mother, or the child has been damaged emotionally at an early stage and is full of bewildering and frightening ambivalent feelings towards the mother that cannot be expressed or understood. The feelings emerge as a phobia of something happening to the mother or sometimes another member of the family from some external and uncontrollable force. These are the beginnings of a possibly severe adult obsessional problem which, if acute, could persist throughout life. The most useful remedies are often *Argentum nit., Natrum mur., Kali. carb., Calcarea,* and *Lycopodium.*

The Passive Child

These children are often thought to be lazy which is not the case. They may provoke reactions of irritability felt as pressures by the parents, which heightens the passivity and underlying uncertainties. The commonest cause is quite simply one of temperament and nervousness, where lack of confidence is to the fore. They do not want to do anything or to go anywhere, are quiet, nervous and only seem secure in the home. They agree with and passify others out of fear and to fob off imagined threats and demands, although at other times they can be obstinate and resistant to change, again due to their underlying fears. *Pulsatilla* and *Kali. carb.* are both helpful remedies, as is *Causticum*.

A thorough discussion with the parents about the lack of confidence is essential; especially, the mother, child and doctor should be involved. In most cases, it is helpful when the fears are tackled early, admitted to and shared, understood and not laughed at, so that they can be shown to be distorted; this resolves much of the anxiety. Once the problem has been recognized by the parents and discussed there is nearly always an improvement. As the personality matures, strengthened by the homoeopathic remedies, the child grows in confidence, outlook and often both physical and mental stature.

Tantrums

This is nearly always a sign of underlying nervousness and anxiety. A child of six came to the surgery with a mild eczema problem for the first time recently. The child was noisy, disturbed and crying loudly whilst waiting outside. Once in the consulting room she refused to be examined, cried, fought angrily, smacked the mother and would not co-operate until the grandmother was brought in from the waiting room. The child's level of disturbance was marked, although the parents were very surprised to think that there was anything unusual in her behaviour. The reason for the child's bad temper was quite clear however. She had been investigated on two occasions in hospital for a benign heart murmer and was now terrified of doctors. The behaviour and the aggressiveness was hiding a deep-seated fear of being examined and re-hospitalized again, separated from the parents.

The fact that she was an only child was not particularly relevant, although, lacking siblings, she had only the grandmother to turn to and she used her as an ally to work out some of the fears and for reassurance and comfort, rejecting the mother as the agent of the separations. Remedies such as *Chamomilla, Nux vomica* and *Natrum mur.* all have a place in treatment. *Aconitum* is helpful where there has been a definite aggravation of behaviour through fear, and *Arnica* is indicated for the treatment of a previous stress or shock and for the separation anxiety.

Clumsiness

This can be a worrying problem for parents and may be linked to accident-proneness. The condition may also occur after a prolonged and difficult birth, or one that was very precipitate. In such cases there may be one limb that has a weakness or some degree of spasticity, although not present to any severe and incapacitating degree. In many cases there is no history of such weakness or of a difficult birth, but the child is sensitive to an extreme degree. They are often artistic but lack spatial judgement and aptitude so that whatever is done is done badly. Ask the child to go out to play for a short period before a trip. The child will usually come back having fallen, grazed a knee or torn a trouser seat. When they bring in the milk, in a helpful way, there is a real danger that they will fall and trip, spill the milk, or just by a miracle save it, grazing an elbow in the attempt. They are willing children but they just fail to see some slight obstacle in their path as they rush by and lose their balance. Ask the same child to push the pram or mind the baby for a few minutes and often the child will rush off at speed, putting baby, pram, limb and passers-by at risk. Whatever is tackled, these children are unable to avoid some form of mishap. The best remedies include their constitutional remedy initially, followed by the two most useful remedies for accident-proneness — *Lycopodium* and *Kali. carb.*

Hypochondriasis

This is common in the nervous, timid and frightened child. They fear illness, hospitals, doctors and sickness. Headaches are common as are 'Monday morning tummy aches'. The least cramp or pain is translated into an illness or given a medical diagnosis — usually picked up from an adult in the family who has implanted the symptoms in the young mind. Often one of the parents has a chronic problem, not infrequently a psychological one, or a grandparent or an aunt has been talking too much about their symptoms and medications, their doctor and their remedies. All of this can put ideas and phantasies into a sensitive and suggestible infant who, because of weak and immature identity patterns, takes on the thoughts, ideas and preoccupations of the sick adult.

The underlying reason is often that the child cannot relate to those of its own age, so that play is weak and too much time is spent with adults. Because their play is unsustained, they do not take part in the usual 'doctor, nurse, hospital' games which help to master anxiety about illness and mortality within the framework of normal play. They become pseudo-adults, full of implanted adult symptoms, problems and attitudes which in the end stunt real development and maturity. The major remedies are often *Lycopodium, Silicea, Pulsatilla* and *Natrum mur.*, and all of these may have a part to play in the treatment. In addition, the family as a whole may need to be seen and even require some counselling in order to take the pressure off the susceptible child.

Physical Symptoms and Recurrent Illness

There are always some physical symptoms accompanying the nervous anxiety of the insecure child. These are very common in the surgery because what is complained of rarely responds satisfactorily and predictably to the conventional approach, because of the underlying emotional component always present. Sedatives, antibiotics, tranquillizers and steroid creams are all tried and, for the majority, the response is unsatisfactory. There may be some relief of symptoms on a temporary basis only, but all too often there is no complete cure. The young patient is soon back in the surgery with the mother, with the same or other problems after a week or two.

Typical problems are asthma, with wheezing and shortness of breath, aggravated by any unusual happening, change of pattern or stress. Migraines and sick headaches are also common, often worse on a Monday morning and better during the holiday period. The headaches tend to be atypical, to vary in position and in intensity and all investigations usually only serve to heighten anxiety in the child and fail to come up with any reasonable cause for the headaches.

Eczema is common from the very first few weeks of life onwards. There is often a similar problem in one of the parents and although the eczema seems to have an allergic base to it, the results of skin tests often show a multitude of possible allergic factors which cannot be used in practise as treatment. An exclusion diet rarely gives any really satisfactory results either, with cheese and chocolate, the common culprits, taken to excess and giving a degree of improvement in the overall eczema condition by eliminating them from the usual diet. But in general the problems persist and may become chronic or intractable, in particular when steroids have been used for prolonged periods in the young patient.

Other common nervous problems with a physical 'face' to them are recurrent 'nervous' diarrhoea, a fear of soiling, colitis, bed-wetting. 'Tummy ache', if recurrent, may lead to the appendix being removed by surgical intervention in an unwarranted attempt to give a surgical cause to a primarily emotional problem. Car sickness, recurrent colds, chronic catarrh, ear ache, insomnia and lack of concentration are all areas of possible nervous disorders. Above all, fatigue and exhaustion are common, the child having large, dark, purple rings under the eyes as an expression of the lack of sleep, the tension and the anxiety.

In all these cases, the constitutional remedy is required initially, followed by the appropriate remedy for the symptoms in a low potency as soon as the constitutional effect is no longer working vigorously enough or does not hold the individual symptoms. Reassurance, exposure of the underlying problems and fears to the light of day and sharing them with the parents are all part of the homoeopathic approach and cure.

3.

EMOTIONAL PROBLEMS OF THE ADOLESCENT

These difficulties inevitably nearly always centre around the major adolescent problem and preoccupation, namely sexuality. This sexuality is inseparable from the growing ego of the adolescent, and is expressed by the profound concern with things physical — such as weight, health, growth, height, colour, their skin and general appearance. There is nearly always a great preoccupation with sexual matters, involving the whole area of physical relationships. This almost obsessional interest in sexuality is an inevitable aspect of maturation, and is a preparation for it as the adolescent develops from childhood, overcoming primitive, infantile narcissm to establish the mature position of family life. Although the adolescent sexuality is largely masturbatory and narcissistic, it is also essentially 'normal' and basic to adolescent development and experience, much as games and play are to the young child; it acts as an essential aid to mastering anxieties about heterosexuality. During such phantasies the adolescent can extend and explore all or most of their uncertainties, wishes and fears.

In this way, sexuality, phantasies and masturbation help the adolescent to master the world as he sees it. Adolescence is always a time of intensity and often of excess and, naturally, sexuality, like all other relationships, is seen and felt to be both sharp and intense. The great confusion of the adolescent is between sexuality as an expression of purely animal and basic instincts, and sexuality as an act of intimate communion with another loved human being. This latter aspect takes time and maturity to develop because initially sex is conceived totally in terms of the physical and of self-gratification, and not as an act of intimate sharing. There exists, therefore, in the majority of adolescents, a split and a confusion between their higher human and inspired, caring selves and the purely animalistic self, concerned with sex as an instrument of procreation, of self-gratification and of narcissism. Both instincts are inevitably present to some degree, varying with the individual and family attitudes.

This is a time, when both the physical and the emotional aspects of the individual reflect the underlying changes and maturation — adjustments for adult life and an active reproductive life. There are many profound physiological, hormonal and psychological changes occurring and, almost invariably, these are experienced in terms of the major adolescent theme of sexuality. Much of the reason behind such a powerful drive is undoubtedly hormonal in nature, as the drive and the preoccupation are far less or absent altogether when, for reasons of disease or delayed development, the hormonal changes have failed to occur. In such cases, not only is the psychological drive absent, but also the corresponding physical development and the anxieties that go with it.

For many adolescents, there is a sense in the early teens of being unprepared, unsure of how to handle themselves, a sense of being a child in an adult frame which they can neither express or control through lack of experience and the psychological uncertainties.

Problems stem from the new roles, challenges, and responsibilities, that inevitably come with the changes and the growth out of childhood into adolescence. Such changes can easily create new pressures, particularly in the weak, uncertain or unconfident child. These problems occur in school, at work, but above all in relationships, particularly the heterosexual ones. Of course, confusion is never admitted as it is inevitably seen as a symbol of a much dreaded weakness; the cardinal sin of the adolescent, who must at all times be above weakness, vulnerability, fear, tears and illness. When 'weakness' occurs in the form of anxiety, uncertainty or fear, it is often felt to be a terrible blow, a thing of shame, to be hidden and denied, lowering their sense of self-esteem which often is one of the most vulnerable areas of their personality.

Lack of a job or of job-opportunities, is the worst of all possible ordeals for any adolescent, who so much needs the reassurance of money, status, and the confirmation of worth that these bring, as well as the discipline. When there is no coherent job structure, which regular employment can bring, there is a lack of psychological coherance, a lack of identity, and a tendency to compensate for such insecurities by joining any group that accepts them, expressing the loss, frustration, violence and sexuality, often in a direct and anti-social way, by becoming drop-outs or drifting into vandalism or petty crime. The failure of society to recognize these prime adolescent needs, and to plan and to provide for them is at least partly to blame for the very serious rioting and destruction occurring in so many cities in 1981.

Alcoholism, drugs, crime and promiscuity are the main danger areas for the adolescent who is left to his own devices without the reassurance and creativity of a work situation. He is exposed to the suggestibility of the mob and the extremist who seeks to recruit such vulnerable youths into structured, sometimes racist, quasi-political movements, which offer them the promise of status and identity. In this way, the sexual energies are channelled into violence and disorder. Of course, there are some adolescents that react to difficulties and frustrations as among life's challenges, and who find a creative outlet in the service of society in their area. Such teenagers have the capacity and the maturity and usually come from an intact family rather than a deprived background; they have the ability to respond to difficulties positively.

Others are less fortunate, and whilst they do not join the group or the mob, losing themselves in violence and mindless behaviour, they are depressed, lonely, isolated, and experience a deep sense of despair and frustration.

The Main Problems Which Arise and Their Treatment

Depression
This is a very common problem in the adolescent, occurring at any time when there are problems and at times of pressure, often from exams, lack of job opportunities, drug taking, a failure in a relationship or insecurities which prevent their development. The depression may be severe, often suicidal, and there has usually been a trauma or a loss, though not inevitably. Sometimes the depression follows a family pattern or there is a strong hereditary history (miasm). Others develop severe depression following a physical illness, as in the cases of glandular fever, influenza or hepatitis.

Recommended remedies include *Naja, Sepia, Natrum mur.* and the nosode for any acute infective condition that may have precipitated the depression.

Schizoid Illness and Schizophrenia
This is common in the over-sensitive, shy, withdrawn adolescent, often immature, and generally where there is a family history of mental instability associated with a preoccupation with body image and sometimes anorexia nervosa. The body image is commonly severely distorted as is the psyche, so that confusion with others and with their 'body borders', outlines and mind is very vague; there may be considerable uncertainty as to where the self ends and the other person begins. This uncertainty is often rationalized and 'understood' by a complicated pattern of delusional beliefs and convictions, which make

for a bizarreness and a distinct pattern of behaviour; any possibility of normal study or work in this condition is impossible.

Anorexia Nervosa

This problem is common in certain over-sensitive girls, being rare in boys. It is common for there to be a 'fat' member of the family or a relative who has a weight problem and has stimulated the fear and the preoccupation with dieting and weight loss. The periods are usually absent and the body weight may be dangerously low, sometimes below six stones (84lbs), so that the general health is impaired. Vomiting is not uncommon and often self induced, and, like the schizophrenic, there is always a distortion of the body image; delusional beliefs are also frequent. Such distortions lead inevitably to the conviction that they are fat and overweight, however thin they are in reality. No amount of reasoning and pressure can seem to change this self image. Remedies include *Thuja, Natrum mur.* and *Cannabis ind.*

Drugs

These may be used by the adolescent for 'kicks' or 'highs' to create an intense period of exhilaration, excitement, and phantasy. The need for such 'highs' is to escape from the 'lows' or sub-clinical depressions, which are never referred to. There is a flight from working through all the problems of growth, conflict and sexuality. During the drug experience, there may be sex, but it is largely uninvolved and free-wheeling and poses no problems of attachment or of caring. It is a form of flight, often closely allied to violence. Discussion by the family of the underlying levels of openness, communication and sharing needs to be combined with the constitutional remedy and repeated often.

Alcoholism

This state is reached when drinking becomes excessive, compulsive and no longer 'social'. Alcohol is another example of flight into the hazy pleasures of easy talk, easy involvements, relaxation and avoidance. It is often linked with drug taking and violence in this age group and is used, like smoking, as a symbol of adulthood and of maturity. When the adolescent is unsure of himself he needs a prop to give him status and credibility, and this leads in some to addiction, dependence and eventually to alienation from others, except similar teenagers who also have a severe drink problem. Such relationships give little lasting satisfaction, and only create more problems for the developing adolescent. Involvements, communication and any form of closeness are anonymous with little real confidentiality, trust or sharing, so that such involvements fail to stimulate any true maturity, and in fact become a barrier to growth, rather than a stimulus.

Smoking

For many groups of adolescents smoking is the classic symbol of maturity, partly of the parents making because of their own indulgence, and partly because of the media, encouraging the cigarette habit as one associated with relaxation, pleasure, enjoyment and sophistication. At the same time as giving an image of adulthood and of adult sexuality, the cigarette also satisfies and perpetuates the infantile need to have something in the mouth. Because smoking undermines health and vitality, it creates dependence and therefore weakness; it gives an impression of ease rather than true maturity and relaxation — it is basically not a desirable habit for the teenager.

Violence

Violence is another form of 'kicks', similar to drugs, but it involves acting out deeply felt hostilities, resentments and sadistic feelings towards other individuals and towards society in general. It is usually carried out anonymously towards a stranger, or in a group or mob. It may be given a racialist rationale and justification. Of course, nothing is ultimately achieved in terms of personal psychological or spiritual growth, and basically it is self-destructive in its lack of concern, compassion, understanding and caring.

Promiscuity

Promiscuity is the sexual 'kick' given tacit approval because of the wide availability of the Pill, and the acceptance by parents, the pharmaceutical companies and the medical profession of the necessity for it. All of this amounts to a non-spoken, sometimes confused acceptance by the parents and by society that sexuality in the teenager should be controlled by hormonal means rather than risk facing an unwanted pregnancy. There is some truth in these arguments for and rationalizations of easy contraception, but nevertheless many parents, let alone teenagers, are not psychologically ready for the freedom and the permissiveness that the Pill has brought; there is often a lot of confusion and many easy sexual relationships because of it. The sexual 'kick' avoids the problems of emotional involvement and the emphasis is generally on the sexual act, urge, passion, power and possession involved but rarely on the loving, caring and giving aspects.

Adolescent Anxiety States

Inevitably, the major problem areas centre around the development of adult sexuality and the need to adjust to the profound hormonal changes which are part of the shift from childhood to adulthood. When there has been a definite, infantile, traumatic cause for anxiety, these areas of damage tend to re-emerge more acutely in adolescence and emphasize the sexual preoccupations and the inevitable uncertainties.

A healthy adolescent stage of psychological development is prepared for by a healthy childhood and usually a secure infant becomes a secure adolescent. It is not now uncommon to meet adolescent girls of 16 or 17 who are on the Pill with both parents' knowledge and approval and with an open discussion of any problems that may arise. These individuals manage to develop a mature relationship with caring and depth over the years, which often culminates in marriage and a family at the age of 17 or 18. Neither the relationship nor the sexuality is in any way a threat or a problem for them. But sadly, in many ways these adolescents are still the exception, and all too often the parental attitudes are rigid, repressive and Victorian, the adolescent is immature, full of uncertainties and problems concerning relationships, either non-existent or promiscuous, over-intense or lacking any real depth or meaning.

Many of the infantile anxiety states already referred to spill over into the adolescent years, complicated by puberty, the onset of menstruation and the adolescent preoccupation with the body image or appearance as an external symbol of inner anxieties. Such inner problems and struggles within the psyche are often concerned with uncertainty and lack of confidence, emerging as the typical teenage preoccupations with the skin, infected spots and acne, or problems of hair, weight and energy. In some, there is an excessive withdrawal into shyness — normal to many adolescents, but when excessive and with a marked self-consciousness, reflecting underlying problems concerning self-confidence and relationships.

Sexual preoccupation with masturbation and some degree of associated guilt is normal because of the nature of the phantasies and the secrecy of it all. This guilt is usually diminished and kept to acceptable, healthy limits, avoiding damage to the developing personality and confidence by the many intense, small-group discussions which frequently arise, both at school and outside it. In addition, the guilt is lessened by the increasing number of television and phone-in 'chat shows' which have an open and frank discussion about such matters. When there is, nevertheless, an excessive guilt, with withdrawal and a lack of balanced relationships with others of similar age, this is often indicative of an underlying anxiety centred around sexual guilt or a similar problem.

Often there is a rebellion against the home and what it is felt to stand for. Its boundaries and rules are resented as is the adult world of convention, leading to a refusal to conform either at home or at school. Such opposition to the norm is established and expressed externally in various dress and hair styles, depending upon which particular group is being supported at the time. Yet within the anti-society, anti-establishment teenage group, the dress quickly becomes another form of uniform itself and the mores within the peer group concerning 'gear' and permitted behaviour can be even more unbending than those of the adult world which they oppose.

The adolescent is often hypochondriacal and fearful so that he may sometimes go through pseudo-religious phases, wandering in mind, talk and phantasy. When the emotional problems are severe, the whole personality is involved in the disturbance, with a remoteness from reality and a tendency to live in a private, unreal world of imagination with marked rigidity of thinking. The disturbances emerge as obsessional food faddiness, general silent moodiness and sullen, uninterested behaviour that is a source of anxiety to friends and family alike.

The major remedies for such anxiety problems always vary with the individual and his particular problems and symptoms at the time. Some of the most important remedies include *Medusa, Gelsemium, Ignatia, Pulsatilla, Natrum mur.* and *Sepia.*

4.

EMOTIONAL PROBLEMS OF
THE ADULT

The adult problem is one of accepting and adjusting to the responsibilities of later life in all its fullness, and of overcoming the narcissistic attitudes and self-indulgences of infancy and its carry-over into adolescence. Maturity implies an overcoming of such attitudes, so that there can be a giving and a sharing in the fullest possible manner, particularly of oneself — one's feelings and ideas. This is the position of normal maturity, and when it is blocked or interfered with, for whatever reason, emotional problems are likely to occur and emotional illness may eventually develop.

It is also true that such maturity, sublimation and transcendence of the inherent narcissism which is in everyone to a varying degree, is never totally attained or totally static, but like everything that is human, is variable, and at times of strain and pressure, even the most mature adult can revert to the infantile position of self-indulgence, self-protection, and narcissism. Usually in such cases, the lapses are temporary, a sign of strain, and there is a return to attitudes of more concern and thoughtfulness as soon as pressures are lifted.

When there has been an acute trauma in the past, either recently or more remotely, and which is not resolved at the time — for example a traumatic marriage and divorce — these affect all future relationships to some extent; and when such problems are not easily talked about or shared and difficulties have been repressed, then they can be a powerful cause of misunderstanding, distortion, and further problems. Usually when earlier traumas, whatever their cause, have not been adequately dealt with at the time, they re-emerge, often unchanged; the feelings intrude on any relationships of the moment as a natural part of the need to work through unresolved problems.

Menopausal problems occur in men and women alike, often from the late thirties onwards, and are an added stress to the problems of modern living in a pressurized society at a time of insecurity and economic difficulties. Such menopausal pressures are particularly disturbing as they are hormonal and therefore internal, taking place deep within the physiology of the individual. At this time of life, there is a change from a physiology which is primarily geared to an active reproductive cycle to one which is less demanding and less cyclical in form and pattern. Such changes are most clearly seen in the female, in terms of the classic changes in the regularity of the menstrual cycles; but in the male they also occur, and because they are not so clearly expressed may cause a lot of confusion, depression, and a personal crisis of emotions, which is not always obviously linked to the underlying hormonal elements.

In the female there is often a return to more adolescent and infantile patterns of attention-seeking and reassurance behaviour, with a variability in mood and even hysterical instability, based on changing hormonal patterns, with an added demand for reassurance, acceptance and love, all marked by outbursts of emotion and rage.

In the male there are also similar emotional explosions and often ill-understood and confusing feelings, irritability, depression or a reversion to adolescent behaviour with promiscuity, fatigue, acne, all reappearing as an expression of the mixed hormonal and regressional emotional process. Back problems and indigestion may also occur as an expression of the changes and the adjustments being made over a period of several years.

In an ideal situation of the fully mature adult, there are no infantile, blocked attitudes; they are overcome by the quality and the depth of caring and of sharing openness with another person. Such a degree of concern can be stronger than the primitive, underlying, narcissistic attitudes and drives. The commonest emotional problem areas are:

Anxiety and Loss of Confidence
This is nearly always rooted in infancy and based on such basic areas of human emotion as fear, loneliness, avoidance, pride, isolation and traumas. In particular, the traumas occur in the areas of separation, hospitalization, battering and violence, parental separations, physical illness of various types, and usually long, drawn out, chronic problems of ill health. The whole problem of mental illness or subnormality in a parent or sibling can be a major trauma for some, and contribute in a major way to feelings of rejection or sometimes guilt.

In the majority of cases, the anxiety is centred around meeting others, together with feelings of low self-esteem, and a corresponding over-inflation of the esteem of others — their qualities, gifts and successes — all these add to the sense of inadequacy, failure and depression.

Anxiety tends to be a common problem in adults when there has been a closed, rigid upbringing and it tends to reflect old attitudes, fears and anxieties of the parents or of an earlier generation, so that these ideals, attitudes and areas of approval and disapproval still influence the adults many years after their sphere of influence upon the child. The anxiety felt is always about the impressions that they make on others, reflecting the importance of outside opinions, esteem, admiration or lack of it, which is so often the key to their self-confidence. In any social situation, these individuals are always under pressure, and inevitably there is a tendency for competitiveness and envy to occur because of their own harsh judgement of themselves. Their lack of confidence is in proportion to their inflated opinions of others and to their fears of rejection. But in many ways, they themselves are their own worst enemies and the cause of most of their pain and suffering.

Depression

Like anxiety, to which it is closely related, depression is one of the most common adult problems, particularly in the 40-year age group. It is common in both men and women and at all ages, and can be either long-standing and chronic — the so-called endogenous depression — or it may be a reaction to and precipitated by a situation or an event, with a sense of failure and futility — the reactive depressions. In fact, there are no clear-cut differentiating features and both are often associated and can occur together.

In many cases, the depression is not always clearly expressed as a depressive problem, and it may often be masked by other apparent problems. Some of the common problems which occur and which mask depression are alcoholism, backache, migraines, obesity, excess smoking, gambling and the need for 'kicks'; promiscuity and compulsive affairs in the 40-year old, indigestion, marital irritability and tensions, frequent visits to the doctor with a multitude of minor and often obscure complaints. A further factor is that the symptoms are usually treated by a mixture of sedatives, tranquillizers and anti-depressants, which often either fail to help, or more commonly add to the feelings of anxiety and depression by causing a sense of fatigue, confusion and sometimes of dependency on the prescribed drugs.

Agoraphobia

This is the common female phobic problem in the 30- to 40-year-olds, and is much more rare in the male. The fear covers a loss of confidence and often the unconscious urge to break away from an intolerable, unhappy and frustrating situation where there is ambivalence; the fear of breaking out as a person, however, and of changing an attitude — for example of passivity — is acute and usually arises in a tense family or marital situation, (though this may not be acknowledged). In general, such attitudes are long-standing, and have often been covered by a stream of obscure and trivial complaints, investigated over the years without a positive outcome.

Psychosomatic Problems

Hypertension, coronary illness and heart attacks; asthma, psoriasis, eczema, allergies, headaches and migraines; ulcers (peptic and duodenal) obesity and excess smoking are all common physical problems, which often have an emotional basis. When stresses of modern living are great, in particular in the overworked executive who is under pressure because of cuts, threats of redundancy and possibly marital tensions, such physical problems are quite likely to arise. All too often the contributing factors are the self-made stresses of the self-made man, with lack of exercise, wrong thinking and wrong values, working for a system, without spiritual values, aims or depth. When there is a family history of psychosomatic problems, as mentioned above, this naturally adds to the intensity of the problem and to the difficulty of its cure.

Paranoid Illness

This is more commonly a male illness, usually occurring in middle age, and of unknown origin. The background is usually one of a rigid, repressive control of the developing personality and attitudes, especially where the underlying personality is obsessionally isolated from others. Latent or unexpressed homosexuality is a common source of anxiety and frequently becomes a feature of the delusions and beliefs. Others are frequently felt to be either accusing or plotting to discredit the individual in some way, often by false accusations of homosexual interests and intentions at some time during the delusions. Attitudes towards women are mistrustful and sado-masochistic, yet at the same time it is other men who are often felt to be the enemy in one form or other.

Schizophrenia is a more common problem, especially of the young adult, occurring in both sexes.

For a detailed guide to the treatment and remedies of the adult psychological problems, see the chapter sections as indexed. In all cases, homoeopathy is concerned with lessening tension and depression, whatever the adult problem. It is important to keep in mind that for any relationship to flourish there must be a sharing and a communication which homoeopathy can facilitate. However, it can not provide the dialogue itself, and for everyone who has an emotional problem, sharing, openness, explanation and discussion of underlying feelings are essential at the same time as the homoeopathic treatment.

5.

EMOTIONAL PROBLEMS OF
THE ELDERLY

Whatever the age group of the person, all living is a time for constant adaptation to changes of both a physiological and a psychological nature. This is especially true of the elderly who have to adapt once again to a different phase of activity with a different physiology and different mental attitudes and often a new feeling within. For the majority, this is a period of quiet, less active and more restricted life, both physically, and often financially, as reserves of physical energy and strengths wind down to some extent. Often there is involvement, usually more indirectly, depending on the interests and experiences of the individual but in general this a time for more reflection and a less dramatic life pattern is the rule.

For others, however, in spite of the inevitable physiological reductions in strength, it is also a period of enthusiasm, often at a literary or artistic level, with gifts, abilities and output still at a peak. Unless there is a period of physical illness, depression or overwhelming loss, these creative outputs continue and the quality of work, in spite of disabilities — even blindness, severe arthritis or deafness — may be considerable. Many show great courage, in spite of problems and physical limitations, with a humour and an attitude of 'refusal to yield', which is admirable. When loneliness, depression or severe physical disabilities with pain are not problems, there is very often a warmth and joy — usually with a story to tell — reflecting deep feelings of thanks and peace as well as humour for their experiences of life — however difficult they may have been at certain periods.

At all ages there has to be a coming to terms with ageing, with immortality and with death. This is particularly important for the older person, so that death and dying may be seen as part of a natural life process, to be shared and acknowledged within the relationship of the couple and not denied or glossed over, nor morbidly indulged in either. It is unfortunate, but common, to see how many couples, apparently close and often church-goers, are quite unable to acknowledge the inevitability of death, and when there is in reality a severe or terminal illness, that it is neither shared nor acknowledged. An experience which is so fundamental and which could add depth, meaning and poignancy to their lives is completely denied and not discussed.

The Commonest Emotional Problems and Some Homoeopathic Remedies

Depression, Fear of Dependency, Retirement and of Death

Ultimately such fears of old age reflect fears of death itself and are usually felt as an anxiety which varies in degree and depth. There is a fear of being a nuisance, a burden, useless, unable to cope, unwanted and lonely. This fear of death is always present, a source of anxiety as the body is felt to decline, and is always worsened by depression or pain, leading to agitation, particularly in an over-anxious personality. For such states of agitation and fear the remedies *Lycopodium, Arsenicum* and *Sepia* are valuable. The death of a colleague and of contemporaries, adds to this awareness of the finiteness of things and of immortality. In some, particularly in a depressive, lonely state, there is considerable agitation felt with a tendency to heightened anxiety and confusion. When this happens, *Sepia* and *Natrum mur.* are particularly helpful.

Confusional States with Loss of Memory

The commonest causes are of a physical illness with an infective illness or when the blood pressure is raised. Sometimes it is a consequence of such illness from the side effects of drugs or antibiotics used when there is a sensitivity to them. Stress, isolation, a change of home and environment and senility are all factors. The cause is often obscure and it may follow a shock or a loss, perhaps of a distant friend or relative. Isolation and deafness can be common causes as can blindness — in one form or another, especially from developing cataract. The condition may also occur after a stroke, or during a stay in a nursing home or hospital. There is usually an unfamiliar environment with resulting fear, anxiety and confusion. The remedies to be considered include *Cannabis sat., Natrum mur., Baryta carb., Tuberculinum bov., Belladonna,* and in severe cases *Stramonium.*

Anxiety States

These are nearly always associated with a loss of confidence, fear and isolation. Insomnia is frequent, with often a poor diet, tension and insecurity. It is not uncommon for constipation to be a worry and with any long-standing tendency to over-worry and to distort anxiety easily takes a hold over the person and may overwhelm him. When severe, it leads to agitation, shaking and an increase of general body tone and tension adding to the anxiety and frequent depression.

Delusional States
These occur when there is a combination of a rigid obsessional personality, hypochondriasis and isolation, sometimes associated with an infection of the chest or intestines, either with or without a raised temperature and often diarrhoea, constipation or a mixture of both. Ideas of reference easily develop as the phantasy world takes over that of reality and there is misinterpretation of noise, and of the motives and actions of others, particularly neighbours. In general, specialized help is required to diagnose and to treat the problem and any underlying physical illness.

Hypochondriasis
This is frequent and occurs particularly when there is a rigid, obsessional personality structure, centred around bowel movement with associated melancholia, agitation and depression. *Sepia* is often invaluable.

Lack of Confidence
This is common in some elderly people who are unable to reach a creative position in their lives or who are not prepared for old age. They feel out of touch with things and life in general, undervalued and of no worth. This often reflects their own attitudes of masochism and self-criticism, and the destructive attitudes in many areas of their lives and relationships.

Further Points Concerning Anxiety States in the Elderly
These are common and a major problem is the fear of dependence, of being paralyzed, becoming a total invalid and generally of being unable to cope on their own. A similar fear is that of being hospitalized or put into an institution and also of being a burden to the family, particularly if incapacitated in any way. Often there is agitation and fearfulness related to some problematic situation which needs to be dealt with and which is usually quite simple and straight forward when clarified. Not uncommonly, some maintenance work needs to be carried out, or the house must be sold when the elderly person is unable to live on his own any more.

Where there is senility, loss of memory or confusion, the problems are always aggravated. *Baryta carb.* and *Sulphur* are often useful for such states of mind where there is agitation and a mixture of fear and anxiety. A reduction in eyesight and hearing, adds to the problems and is an additional factor in the confusion and muddle. It is always essential to correct the physical problems as well as the underlying psychological ones. An on-going contact is essential for the elderly; they need input and stimulation to lessen the inevitable effects of ageing, isolation and withdrawal from or by others.

The common and excessive worry about bowel action and bowel habits, especially constipation, may not only be a physical problem but part of an obsessional, almost delusional concern. There may be similar problems with other organs, particularly where there is any tendency to weakness of or lack of control over bladder function. Both *Lycopodium* and *Causticum* can help with such areas of weakness as well as with anxiety. In others, there is agitation, an inability to relax, clumsiness, confusion of thought and depression which need support and help from the family to give confidence again and help lessen the depression.

Often the anxiety problem is not due to senility or to confusion but more to an over-active mind that just cannot wind down. They have spent their lives worrying over something — the future, money, health — and this is just a continuation of these earlier fears and the basic personality. Friends or family often confirm that such personalities were worrying and insecure at the age of 20, and later at 40, and at 80 they are still just the same, only the problem areas have changed somewhat. It is not uncommon to also find that the constitutional remedy that was effective at 20 is just as effective later in life, although the exact prescription and remedy always depends upon the individual, his symptoms and the total picture; this is always the case in the homoeopathic approach, whatever the age of the patient.

6.

ANXIETY

From infancy onwards, anxiety in some degree is familiar to everyone, and is the commonest of emotional disturbances. For most people, it is of passing significance only, with an awareness of heightened tensions and body tone, a sense of excitement, and apprehension in an unfamiliar situation, which is felt to be a threat to security because it is new and of uncertain outcome.

Anxiety may precede an 'event', such as giving a speech, an examination, interview, sports day, or a first night. Sometimes changing schools is a nightmare for both child and parent, the degree of tension depending upon the individual's personality and make-up. Usually the anxiety ends after the event and there is an immediate relief of tension and fear, sometimes built up over a period of weeks.

For many people, giving a good impression is the key to being approved of, loved and accepted. Ultimately this goes back to infantile needs to please and win over the parents, who must often be made to feel proud of their children, impressed and entertained, in order that the child is certain of love and approval. Failure is a great threat because it may lead to parental disappointment, rejection and criticism, loss of esteem and admiration. Although this is usually short-lasting, in some people there is a constant need to be admired and approved of to ensure acceptance from both parents and parental figures.

Any everyday 'happening' may trigger off anxiety, from a wedding reception to a visit to the dentist, whenever it has an importance or emotional significance. The cause of anxiety is nearly always the same — a situation either occurs or is created where there is a threat of disapproval or criticism by others, felt to be superior in position, age, intelligence and experience. This recreates the situation of parental criticism towards the child, and in an insecure person, this sparks off anxiety. Such anxiety is always immature, because it re-establishes the infantile situation of dependency and vulnerability. It is wasteful of vital energy, serving no real and useful purpose in reality, compulsively creating a negative situation which puts the individual at a disadvantage and in an inferior role; the individual overinflates others at the expense of his own qualities and strengths. Such anxiety empties the individual of all vitality, sense of value and achievement, and the more frequently this happens, the worse the draining and damaging effects.

It is helpful at this point to pause in this general discussion of anxiety and to look more closely at some of the personality profiles of the major remedies where anxiety is marked, and where such behavioural patterns indicate the remedy.

Personality Profiles of Some of the Major (polychrest) Remedies

When there is a severe problem of anticipatory anxiety, the remedy of choice is often *Lycopodium* extracted from club moss; it is linked with strong symptoms of obsessional anticipatory anxiety to a degree which can weaken the most able and gifted personality, turning ability to trembling fear, insomnia, collapse and exhaustion. It is one of the broadest and deepest-acting of all the anxiety remedies — an inert powder in its unprepared form, which flashes brightly when ignited. This feature encompasses many of the typical *Lycopodium* characteristics. There is a combination of nervous excitement and intelligence in flashes, which comes and goes, like everything that is *Lycopodium*. This includes the ability to concentrate, which is always sporadic, and is typified by the butterfly mind which settles at nothing; hence the patient's common complaint of a poor memory, because he is never concentrating long enough to retain and remember information. The inertness of the original substance is marked, linking up with chronic fatigue, tiredness and a constant fear of any new situation.

Much of the marked lack of confidence comes from this intrinsic restlessness, so that such individuals can never really gain in a new experience or relationship. They are always running away or ahead, feeling threatened, so that they fail to develop on or to solidly integrate, many of their primal and basic experiences in life. Almost anything is seen as a threat or a demand, and they dread failure. Typically, they bury themselves in the safety of intellectual pursuits, eschewing competitive sport or contact with others where there is a risk of failure. They are the 'boffins' or 'ideas men', brilliant yet restless, never really relaxed and always on the move — fidgety, both mentally and physically.

Because of their haste to finish with the task in hand, and their need to get away — to be somewhere else, or to do something else — they live in the future, never in the present, cannot be nailed down to a commitment and are always one step ahead. They live in the future, yet it is the future that is feared and dreaded at all costs, particularly when they may be questioned or find themselves the centre of attention. Their performance on the day is usually adequate, but lacks lustre since they long so much to be elsewhere and finished — away. Another emotional remedy is also restless, namely *Arsenicum;* however, this differs in that many of the severe obsessional qualities and drive for success and achievement are lacking in the typical personality requiring *Lycopodium.*

In others, there need be no particular event to trigger anxiety. Anxiety in such cases is stimulated by a change in the pattern of the everyday routine which is resented. A weekend visitor is felt to be an intruder, taking away the partner or leisure time, making demands and creating problems when there is already enough to cope with. Such visits or demands may be experienced as an intruding younger sibling who takes away the mother and, through his demand for attention, threatens to deprive the older child of her. Anxiety in these personalities is related to the re-emergence of strong infantile hostility. Such hostility is feared because it may be overwhelming, but also because it may alienate them from the mother and make them unpopular. Fear of change is characteristic of a rigid personality make-up, and particularly *Natrum mur.* has this quality, being basically a preservative, and a hardener of both tissues and attitudes. This accounts for the typical lack of flexibility, the strong drive to preserve the established and the familiar and the ruthless opposition to intrusion and change.

Sodium chloride or common salt in potency, as *Natrum mur.,* is one of the deepest-acting homoeopathic remedies. The constitutional characteristic of the remedy is the need to control oneself, and the avoidance of sympathy and consolation in any form due to the fear of breaking down and giving way to weakness. There is a stiff upper-lip attitude in all circumstances, and these personalities abhor any form of attention and fuss. They quickly show their lack of control in any situation of illness or pressure, which leaves them feeling inadequate and irritable — mainly with themselves, but also with others. In a stress situation there is a change, and extreme emotionability, with a sudden switch from tears of concern or grief to laughter and then irritability. They are over-sensitive, and cannot relax whatever the situation, moving about in their thought-processes in a haphazard way, and as restless in their bodies. Generally they are never fully at ease in any social situation, wherever they are.

In other personalities the anxiety is related to excessive shyness and the fear of making a 'show', becoming unduly excited or emotional with loss of control. Such fears and anxieties are really a thin cloak to hide the enormous unconscious drive to carry out and express what they most fear — namely making an 'exhibition of themselves'. There is a constant need to do this, whatever the situation, so that they constantly recreate a mixture of shame and drawing attention to themselves, the shyness a mixture of shame, guilt, and a compulsive need to be in the limelight.

When anxiety is fixed and lasting, not related to any particular event, seemingly without reason and not responding to simple common sense measures of reassurance and encouragement, then a situation is present which threatens the security and normal life of the individual and family. In most cases, treatment is required to prevent a chronic state developing. For the majority, homoeopathy is the safest and most efficient way of treating and resolving such problems.

The most common symptoms of lasting anxiety are a sense of malaise, of being uncomfortable and ill at ease. This sense of uneasiness, together with a vague sense of free-floating and unrelated tension, heightens the anxiety. Feelings of oppression and restlessness are common and such symptoms are usually felt in either the chest or abdomen, and often misinterpreted as signs of heart trouble, cancer, an ulcer, or confirming some hypochondriacal fear. Often there is nausea, with a loss of appetite, heartburn, sometimes diarrhoea, or the frequent passing of water. Others eat compulsively in any situation when they feel anxious, insecure or threatened. Such excesses carry their own problems of pain, flatulence, discomfort, obesity and nausea, creating an additional matter for concern. Not infrequently , breathing is also affected, becoming irregular, often with overbreathing, sometimes sighing in type. If prolonged, it may lead to fainting attacks, sometimes to tetany, when there are shaking attacks of the limbs, to the consternation of both patient and family. All of these symptoms will confirm that something is deeply wrong, perhaps incurable. Often there is a conviction that either the condition has been misdiagnosed, or that the diagnosis is being kept a secret by the doctors. The other common symptom is of a great intolerance of heat or stuffiness in any form, provoking clammy feelings and palpitations, sometimes collapse. Such symptoms of heat intolerance and the need for fresh air are an indication for a prescription of *Pulsatilla*, the windflower, anenome, or flower of change.

Pulsatilla is well known as a remedy for female complaints, but it is often less well appreciated that this is also very effective in the male when the primary characteristics of the remedy are present. *Pulsatilla* anxiety is of an irritable, peeved type in a personality that is outwardly passive and apparently easily led. In a situation at home, however, where they feel more sure, they can be very different, both difficult and contradictory. The tendency to be changeable is the great characteristic of the remedy, and it is true for every aspect of their personality. The anxiety itself is equally changeable, one moment depressive, then hysterical and emotional — a mixture of tears and laughter — one minute confident, and then collapsing under some imagined insult. They are always dependent people, better for sympathy and consolation. Because of their sense of insecurity, these individuals are not good with their own company, easily becoming fearful or depressed alone, because their self-image in their own mind is low; basically they have little interest in their own company and often few real interests. Their overwhelming need is for approval, to be liked, agreed with, the basic personality constantly needing to be bolstered by others, which adds considerably to their extreme vulnerability.

There is also another type of personality make-up which is commonly seen. Here there is a marked sense of failure, rejection, inadequacy, such as may follow the ending of a relationship, or its break-down. This can sometimes lead to a permanent state of anxiety. The underlying mechanism is one of extreme feelings of rage and resentment at any criticism or rejection, sometimes directed at the self for having failed, or not been able to resolve all the problems which contributed to the ending. There are unrealistic demands made upon the self to be omnipotent, to be able to resolve all things, all problems, and to reach impossible standards of either loving, understanding, or forgiveness. They are doomed to perpetual feelings of failure, and are never satisfied or fulfilled. Because they are so over-critical in their attitudes to themselves and others, they are often very difficult people to live with. The tendency to be over-critical, over-zealous, to aim for unrealistically high standards is typical of the *Nux vomica* type of problem, and is an indication for the remedy.

Nux vomica takes its origin from the poison nut strychnine, and throughout its actions, this origin exerts its influences. This is particularly noticeable in the emotional field, with the typical tendencies to spasm and increased irritability. The basic personality is, first of all, irritable and aggressive in type, with short bursts of heat, rage and resentment that flares up and just as quickly cools down and is over. *Nux vomica* types are over-sensitive to everything — the least noise, draught or bright light irritates and provokes feeling of intolerance. This varies with age from outbursts of temper tantrums in the child, falling down and screaming with rage in the street and stamping the feet on the pavement, or a more controlled and limited outburst. The adolescent and adult can be quite impulsive and violent, having a short fuse with poor self-control, whatever the provocation. They have bursts of energy, spasms of ambition, and in general everything has this tendency to sudden excess and unreasonableness. Nothing is ever done moderately or in a natural, quiet, rhythmic way. This inevitably leads to periods of tiredness and exhaustion, a tendency to indulge in alcoholic stimulants, again excessively and spasmodically, with the inevitable consequences for health. Strychnine in its unprepared form is an extreme form of excitant, and this type of personality can never delegate responsibility, needing to control matters because of their basic distrust of others. At night they rarely sleep well or deeply, and this only serves to increase their misery, irritability and fatigue.

Sometimes confidence is lacking in an unduly sensitive person, anxious to please, and wanting company. They are of pleasing, attractive and lively disposition, popular and out-going, but suffering intently at the least slight or joking criticism. Such a person may require *Phosphorus* in its homoeopathic remedy form, in order to cope with underlying insecurities and anxieties.

Phosphorus, like *Lycopodium*, is quite an inert substance until it is thrown into contact with one of the basic elements of nature, when it explodes with great force and bursts into flames. This quality of the 'mother-remedy' explains the personality for which it is indicated. There is a combination of inertness and exhaustion; the least physical or mental effort exhausts, contrasting with an equally violent tendency to flare up into passionate, impulsive rages and, having flared up, to sink back into inert exhaustion. The very brightness of their personality, accounts for the popularity of these types.

Such a make-up has an enormous need for reassurance, and in the surgery they tend to keep their eyes fixed on the doctor, reflecting their fear of the outcome. This fearfulness is characteristic; they are typically always nervous of something happening. The extreme sensitivity of this personality is seen whenever there is a change of atmospheric pressure; then excitement or restlessness build up, as with the approach of thunder or a storm. This link with the elements and the characteristic sensitivity may relate to the intolerance of music, especially the piano, which seems to irritate profoundly. A similar sensitivity, to the point of apparent pain, is sometimes seen in certain animals who are threatened and disturbed by music, and equally restless and disturbed when there is about to be a storm or change in the weather. The least change in the moisture content of the atmosphere excites or irritates at either a physical or emotional level, as if the *Phosphorus* type is ready to burst into flames, like the mother substance itself.

Arsenicum alb. is indicated for the perfectionist who experiences anxiety because he consistently takes on too much, always overstretching himself. There is a compulsive need to overextend, to the point of exhaustion and ill health — as if to impress or placate some internal god or parent-figure, who demands great personal sacrifices from the individual all the time in terms of activity and output. Naturally, such excesses have to be paid for in terms of the quality of life, peace of mind and happiness. To placate and please others is the rule; they cannot say no, and seem caught up in a vicious circle of never stopping, because they 'must push on'. All of this is coupled with the terror of failure, loss of esteem and of humiliation. Love is indirectly expressed to those near them through this activity, often misunderstood, and they fail to understand why so often it leads to isolation and to losing the very thing which they most desire — namely, love and appreciation, acceptance by those around them.

Normal Fears and Anxieties

These are feelings appropriate to a given situation and relating to the physiological release of adrenalin and energy, in preparation for a coming challenge. The sense of anticipation may resemble pathological anxiety, but is much more limited in its boundaries, and not so excessive and overwhelming as the typical anxiety state. There is also far more awareness of being in a state of buoyant anticipation and tension — a mixture of excitement and challenge, rather than the opposite state of unrelated, free-floating anxiety. The true anxiety state is related to excessive feelings, out of place to the situation and inappropriate to the degree of demand made upon the individual.

We are all faced with normal fears and anxieties every day of our lives. Normal fear is a helpful warning reaction, an essential preparation for the resolution of the task in question. Such fear indicates that the body is ready and geared up to meet the challenge. The absence of normal fear with a totally negative reaction, a flatness, or emotional vacuum, would seriously impede the individual from being at his peak when dealing with a difficult task. In some situations, depending upon the individual personality and make-up, anxiety may accompany the normal heightened awareness and anticipatory tone, but such severe reactions are usually only short-lived and do not constitute an illness.

This experience of normal heightened tone or normal anxiety before an event, fades normally once it has started, quickly giving way to a sense of relief and relaxation and often positive pleasure, as the earlier fears and phantasies are seen to be based on distortion, so that a sense of achievement replaces the fear.

In some cases there may be the need for some reassurance afterwards — was it alright?, how did it go?, but such needs are only of a temporary nature, and fall within normal limits of all individuals needing a degree of feed-back and reassurance.

Depressive anxiety is present when the quality of emotion experienced is primarily depressive in type. There is a profound sense of failure, inadequacy, shame and guilt, contributing to the sense of tension which is rarely absent. Underlying phantasies of rage, revenge and destructiveness predominate, and emerge as dreams of desolation, war, or persecution. Such dreams often reflect revenge phantasies directed at a sibling or sibling-figure, or sometimes an adult figure in the dream reflects ambivalence towards a parental image. To some extent, the underlying rage and persecution also occurs in work and social relationships, and it is rare for the dreams not to also reflect and mirror everyday happenings and injustices. Such commonplace, everyday problems can lead to a sense of alienation and rejection, adding further to depression and feelings of failure. Quite often, there has been a bout of verbal aggression, and it is not uncommon to find that prior to depressive anxiety, there has been a period of being particularly outspoken. Such plain speaking has sometimes occured during a 'good' or 'high' period, when there has been a 'putting in place' and a dotting of the i's and t's.

Sometimes there is an overwhelming need to stay in the home, in a vain attempt to find security from inner fear and doubt. There is a constant preoccupation with others and what they are thinking about them, and fear that any thoughts and comments must inevitably be unfavourable. There is a fear of being natural when with others. High standards are frequently set, and often there is undue emphasis on success, rather than being natural and oneself. All of this easily leads to an exaggerated sense of self-criticism, so that work and dealings with people become pressurized, competitive situations at all times, and just cannot be faced. Insomnia is frequent, and there may be oppressive nightmares, full of hostile figures, reflecting the underlying aggressive phantasies, and the unconscious tendency to be self-critical and destructive.

Causes and Onset

Often there has been an imagined failure, such as loss of a potential job opportunity, a promotion check, failure to interview well for a new post. In others, it follows a redundancy, and is particular in the 40-year age group, when there is an increased tendency to depressive anxiety. But the problem may occur at any time from early adolescence. There are no self-destructive tendencies, but such phantasies may occur as part of the general morbidity, and the idea of getting away from it all, or as a means of avoiding some new and challenging situation, which should be dealt with in a realistic way. Failure to take advantage of opportunities as they arise, and to often destroy the possibility of success and achievement are part of the reason for underlying guilt feelings. Sometimes much earlier infantile problems of fear, separation and loss come to the surface again. This may happen particularly when there is a temporary separation of husband and wife for work reasons, either partner having to work away for a few weeks or months; a threatening situation may be created while a house is being sold or a new one found. Such problems are really recreations of infantile insecurities as much as at a 'reality' level.

Concealed Depressive Anxiety
Concealed or 'smiling' depression occurs when depressive anxiety is bottled up and denied, so that problems and worries are not openly shared, and tend to fester and grow into unreal proportions. There is a tendency for them to re-emerge as physical symptoms; duodenal ulcer, migraines, chronic back pain, recurrent colds, and various psycho-somatic problems can take the place of underlying depressive anxiety, and a smiling 'fixed' face is given to the world. To the family and friends the patient may appear normal and well, much the same as usual. There seems to be nothing much wrong. This does not imply that the family is particularly insensitive, rather that there has been little sharing of true feelings over the years and there has been some reluctance to trust and be open within the family. Such concealed smiling depression may be dangerous, particularly because it can so easily go unnoticed, and there may be a sudden suicidal attempt in a move to draw attention to underlying despair.

Remedies for a Concealed (Smiling) Anxiety State

1) *Arsenicum*
There is the typical picture of the *Arsenicum* make-up as already described. The face is often fixed in a rigid smile which easily becomes a grimace, and is more of a mask than any true expression of joy or relaxation and contentment. Inflexibility with a tendency to deny problems is generally characteristic of the make-up where this remedy is indicated, and this same inflexibility is present in the outer gestures and mannerisms. The make-up of the personality is such that he does not readily and easily confide, and usually prefers to make an outward show of normality.

2) *Causticum*
Timid, nervous, fearful, particularly of the dark, with nervous diarrhoea often a severe problem (as with *Gelsemium*). The smile and outward charm is part of the marked sympathy which is so characteristic of this remedy and which reflects the most intense concern of these types for the pain and suffering of others. Recurrent warts are nearly always present. Tension in the throat, jaw or neck area is common, and all symptoms are worse at twilight.

3) *Gelsemium*
This remedy is associated with intense anxiety, particularly for the future (*Lycopodium*) and nervous diarrhoea (*Causticum, Argent. nit.*). Basically, these individuals want peace and quiet and, above all, not to be disturbed. The smile of outward apparent calm is to discourage others from disturbing them and increasing their anxiety.

4) *Phosphorus*
This remedy is linked with extreme nervousness and sensitivity, always worse at twilight (*Causticum*) and also aggravated by music and thunder (*Sepia*). Constant reassurance is needed hence their 'niceness' and popularity, needing above all to be liked and loved. The severe nervousness of *Phosphorus* types is often hidden beneath their need of others and of social contact.

5) *Natrum mur.*
In general, anxiety is concealed quite consciously because of the need at all costs to avoid the sympathy and concern of others, which is experienced as intolerable interference, and to prevent worsening the underlying state by a heightening of tension.

Agitated Anxiety
This is more common in older age groups, although it can occur in middle age. It is often the sign of an impending nervous breakdown, as a combination of restless self-reproach and anxiety becomes over-whelming. Physically, the face is flushed, and there is an inability to rest or relax. Agitation may be severe, both mentally and physically, with tremor and twitching of the feet, knees, legs and arms to an alarming and uncontrollable degree. There is a tendency to sweat and the person looks care-worn and older than his or her years, introverted and lonely, preoccupied, often barely attentive. The individual tends to be aware of only one thing—his inability to sleep or relax. Sometimes it occurs after an attack of influenza, or a prolonged period of tranquillizers.

Usually the basic make-up is rigid and obsessional, sometimes hypochondriacal too. There is a fear of fear itself, a sense of helpless failure. Sometimes such a reaction follows a loss, precipitating a fear reaction, but in most cases the cause is obscure, and the anxiety long-standing.

Recommended Remedies for Agitated Anxiety States

1) *Arsenicum*
One of the major remedies for an agitated state of mind, varying from agitated anxiety to agitated states of depression. See the earlier general section for a complete personality profile, but note that one of the major diagnostic features is the need for heat, and the tendency to be chilly and overdressed on the warmest summer day.

2) *Borax*
There is a state of fidgety nervous anxiety, specifically worse for any form of downward or forward motion — particularly the movement of a rocking chair, swing, going down stairs or through air-pockets when flying. All the above movements provoke severe vertigo and anxiety.

3) *Bryonia*
There is a combination of irritability and agitated anxiety, in spite of the fact that all symptoms are worse for movement. Stitch-like pains are diagnostic as well as chest weakness, so that a dry nervous cough is often present.

4) *Calcarea*
Chilly weakness and 'unhealthy' fatness, quite unable to relax or to stop obsessional pointless movement and agitation.

5) *Iodum*
There is a restless anxiety that something is about to happen; the individual is irritable and impulsive to the point of violence and there is a need to act or do something without delay. They are markedly warm-blooded and only find comfort in a cool room (*Pulsatilla*). There is canine hunger and often the only relief comes from eating or from movement in fresh air.

Phobic Anxiety States
The main problem of individuals suffering from this type of anxiety is one of being dominated by fear. They are always insecure, often fearful

of the dark as young children, and troubled by nightmares as adults as in childhood. The underlying personality is that of a weak, fearful, vulnerable and obsessional type easily threatened by any change in the usual pattern. There is often little family security in the early years, and the overall pattern is one of frailty and collapse at the least threat. Because of the anxiety, growth and maturity is subjugated to the domination of fear and the preoccupation with it; normal experiences leading to growth are invariably stunted in the same way as the personality, and often the physique.

There is a sense of being troubled by something, often it is quite nameless and indefinable, seemingly beyond awareness and consciousness, so that the person cannot explain what brings about such a feeling of anxiety and near-terror. There is a fear of everything; the least event can trigger off the phobic reaction, and it is often barely subdued when in bed or at home with the doors locked. Only very gradually can a situation of relaxation and security develop, because of the constant sense of impending disaster, foreboding and superstition. Almost anything can provoke an attack of panic — a letter or bill, even the telephone ringing is a threat, and the thought of meeting anyone other than the closest member of the family is like a torture. They are not, however, confined to the house, or prevented from working, and the fears are just kept sufficiently in check to prevent a total breakdown, in spite of the feeling that everything outside the home is a demand, a threat and a pressure.

Often since childhood the whole of life has been dominated by fear, involving every aspect of living and every relationship. There is a constant fear of being late for appointments, so that such an individual usually comes early just in case something were to hold him up, and is often accompanied on a first visit. During a consultation or any conversation, they tend to be unduly intense and attentive, fearing missing the point, eyes glued on the speaker. Because nothing ever really reassures them, they are often repetitive, demanding and obsessional, and fearful of the doctor, the remedies given, the outcome of treatment, and of it making them worse and not better. The least reaction to the remedy is often taken as a negative sign, at which they look for reassurance that they are not worse or even incurable.

Recommended Remedies for Phobic Anxiety States
See the section on Fears and Phobias for general comments and further details of remedies.

1) *Argentum nit.*
This remedy is linked with typical obsessional-phobic thinking with many compulsive patterns and avoidances — ladders, pavement cracks, or certain dates. Superstition is marked as is the conviction that death is imminent to the point of being obsessed with the thought. Exhaustion and tension are common with always the greatest intolerance of heat of any form (*Pulsatilla, Iodum*). Indigestion, flatulence and a history of peptic ulcer is usually present to some degree, and provoked by the chronic underlying state of tension.

2) *Anacardium*
There is a peculiar hysterical dissociated state linked with this remedy, with many bizarre features and convictions, including the feeling of being followed or having a double (*Baptisia, Petroleum*). There is confusion, a tendency to strong language, and constipation — as if the bowels were blocked by a plug.

3) *Drosera*
There is a restless pattern of silent suspicion and mistrust, with an inclination to drowsiness. Pessimism is marked and a nervous cough or laryngitis is common.

4) *Graphites*
Hesitant indecisiveness is the pattern here in a vulnerable emotional make-up. These personalities are over-sensitive, easily moved to tears and immature. The physical constitution is usually chilly and obese (*Calcarea*). A rather odd, but specific diagnostic symptom is a sensation of having a cobweb over the face and needing to constantly try and brush it away.

Psychosexual Anxieties
These can occur at any age, but they are especially common in the young, particularly the adolescent. The anxiety centres around problems of making contact, meeting others and self-expression — knowing what to say and how to say it. The problem is not directly related to heterosexuality, since when the basic orientation is homosexual, the problems are still present. For the majority, the problem is one of distortion and often overvaluation of the opposite sex, leading to problems of fear, flight, and feelings of inadequacy. Frequently, there has been a failure in childhood in the development of trust and confidence with one of the parents, which has led to the feelings of failure and lack of confidence. There is usually both a desire

for contact and a relationship, at the same time as a marked tendency to withdraw into loneliness and feelings of defeat. Shyness is common, and usually there is an excessive tie to a member of the family.

Such fears are a common adolescent problem, often with sweating and undue shyness in the presence of the opposite sex. Masturbation is always normal in the adolescent, particularly when there are no external relationships to balance and to compensate for growth and the changing hormones. Such phantasy masturbatory relationships are often violent in quality, intense and secret, as well as very exciting. There is a natural, omnipotent, magical quality about such feelings which may create guilt and add to the barrier and the shyness.

Of course, many adolescents are now taking the Pill from the age of 15 onwards, either with or without the consent of the parents, and have commenced a full physical relationship which is sometimes long-standing. This is often discussed openly with the parents and agreement reached as to a contraceptive method. Naturally, the outcome of such an early relationship depends on the maturity of the couple and many other complex factors. But quite often there are no severe problems because of the degree of openness, and in others the parents are there to pick up the pieces should a disaster occur.

Others are less fortunate, and drugs, promiscuity, alcohol, violence and crime may mask problems of inadequacy, and be used to impress and to gain favour, depending upon the background and social group. Some adolescents rush prematurely into an adult world of premature sexuality to hide their fear of it, and as an expression of hostility to what appears to be a hostile, authoritarian, parental society.

In the adult, there may have been a longing for contact since adolescent. Sometimes a contact has been made in the past, and confidence never regained after a hurt, trauma or break-down. In others, the person has been controlled and tied to possessive parents, and has not been strong enough to make the break. A sense of confidence may never have developed, nor a feeling of independence or of the self. Often the earliest childhood relationships were weak, not properly developed, and the child was over-sensitive. When there have been obsessional tendencies, this has created a much more rigid and controlled personality and increased the difficulties, so that any approach to another is over-tense. This excessive control makes for discomfort in the other person, and the stiff, ungainly body movements which frequently occur are an aspect of unconscious body language. Finally, such a move away is inevitably interpreted as a rejection, as a failure, and to mean that they are unlovable and unattractive, particularly to anyone of the opposite sex.

Recommended Remedies for Psychosexual Anxiety States

See the chapter specifically dealing with psychosexual problems.

1) *Lycopodium*

See the general introductory section in this chapter for a profile of the personality characteristics and indications for this remedy. In general, *Lycopodium* is connected with insecurity in all situations, particularly when there is contact with the other sex. In many ways, such a personality takes flight from these encounters through high-flying theories, intellectual pursuits and manoeuvres which maintain a distance from feelings and vulnerability. There are many potency problems and anxieties which add to the difficulties and are in part due to non-involvement; in this way, sexuality tends for much of the time to be at a purely phantasy level.

2) *Silicea*

Weakness, fear and withdrawal characterize this remedy so that there is inevitably a lack of confidence in sexuality and fear of failure in these individuals.

3) *Cyclamen*

This remedy is indicated when the whole personality is paralyzed by feelings of the most inappropriate guilt, (*Staphisagria*). They are easily irritable, and this is often accompanied by a disturbance of vision — particularly a 'flickering' sensation is characteristic.

7.

DEPRESSION AND WITHDRAWAL

Depression is a sense of profound alienation and loneliness with feelings of futility and despair. There is a sense of being cut off from others because of the tendency to withdrawal, which accompanies a sensation of psychological stagnation. Self-isolation, introspection and self-analysis occur as part of the preoccupation with self, and there are increasing feelings of being alone — even when others are there, including the closest members of the family.

There is a sense of flatness, a lack of enthusiasm and zest for living. Nothing really interests the individual with any passion or intensity, everything seems boring and dull, lacking humour and leading to a phlegmatic response to whatever contacts are made. Time seems to pass intolerably slowly, in part because of the awareness of their flatness and lack of response which exasperates and yet cannot be remedied however much they try to 'shake themselves out of it'. There is a marked absence of any buoyant feelings or drive or confidence with others, so that the tendency is to avoid contact, which in turn increases the feelings of defeat and hopelessness.

The self-image is always low, feeling themselves to be dull, hopeless and often without purpose, above all lacking drive physically, sexually or psychologically. Nothing really appeals and everything seems somehow jaded and uninteresting, especially their own mental state. Irritated by others, yet not wanting to be left totally alone is a common feeling — the self-induced isolation from others adding to the depression.

There is a common feeling of having been let down or betrayed by others. But often these others have been idealized, inflated and distorted so that expectations of them were really also inaccurate and unreal. Equally, there is a feeling of being betrayed by their own ideas of themselves and this leads to a sense of imagined failure, defeat and depression and having failed in the eyes of others or in their duties and responsibilities towards them — often another more dependent member of the family.

The frequent preoccupation with ideals, standards and failure is an indication of how the conscience plays a central role in depression; the conscience is often excessive and cruel as can be clearly seen in the self-reproaches and phantasies of self-destruction that are so common.

In fact in depression, contrasting with the overwhelming sense of failure, futility and uselessness of everything, there is an equally powerful preoccupation with standards and ideals — what might have been, and how things were; or how the individual should have been and behaved in a given situation, which itself is an aspect of the self-reproach. In general the feelings of failure are inevitable, because whatever their achievement and whatever their personality, the extremes of the ego-ideal make these achievements a poor second best and lead to inevitable dissatisfaction.

Although fate and others are seen as treating them unfairly, most of the blame is reserved for themselves, and the weight of self-reproach is often heavy for the supposed areas of inadequacy, which only they themselves see as being so serious. What the depressive does not see is the extent of his own self-centredness in his problem; his failures, his hurts, and his hopelessness are central to his condition, but rarely are the feelings of others of any major concern other than to reinforce the individual's inadequacy in this area. This involvement with self is one of the major barriers to resolving and curing the depression.

Sometimes this narcissism becomes extreme and obsessional; the self-involvement is directed at the body and its functions so that there develops a hypochondriacal concern with the body weight, indigestion, loss of appetite and chronic constipation which is a feature of the general sluggishness, physically as well as mentally.

CASE NOTE

A successful business man of 45 came with a depressive problem. He felt flat, without energy or confidence, was in a highly restless and nervous state, and was unable to sleep for more than a few hours before waking in the early hours — about 3.00 a.m. — and being unable to sleep again. His business was almost at a standstill because of economic difficulties and he was obliged to close down several factories and centres with the inevitable redundancies of people he had known for many years and who had always been loyal to him. Such decisions were inevitable, but he kept putting off taking any decisive actions. He was a man who had put all his energies and interests into his business and had nothing outside them to absorb his energy and drive. As long as he was able to expand and develop the business areas he had been happy, but as soon as this was impossible he felt defeated and depressed.

Because of the intense, needing to prove, and irritable aspects of his personality, he was given *Nux vom.* and this was followed by *Kalium carb.* to deal with the lethargy, the despair and the insomnia. The final remedy was *Natrum mur.*, which is used for the tense, nervous, rigid personality traits which he also showed, especially the lack of flexibility in a new situation.

The outcome was a positive one; the sleep improved, he was less obsessed with the problems and decisions which had to be made, and began to reorganize the work areas. The final problem, which homoeopathy could not help with, was the need to find and develop other areas of alternative interest and creativity.

Some Recommended Remedies for General Depression

1) *Natrum mur.*
For emotional, tearful depression. This personality is irritable, of independent make-up, essentially pragmatic and practical, rather than intellectual; always worse for sympathy and consolation. They want to be left alone with their misery.

2) *Lycopodium*
The depression of the intellectual, rather solitary but needs someone in the house, and more social than *Natrum mur.* They are not very emotional people, and their time and energies thinking and making endless speculative plans or possible projects (anticipation). Always worried about the future.

3) *Arsenicum*
Useful when the basic make-up is fussy and obsessional, worried about the past rather than the future. Often exhausted because of their constant fidgety movements and activity. They cannot keep still for a moment — the mind is never at rest because of obsessional thinking and double checking. Even in sleep they toss and turn, and the typical chilliness is partly due to their thin physical build — burning every calorie in endless movements and agitated activity.

4) *Nux vom.*
These individuals are depressed because of some slight or incident or imperfection in the past, leading to a mixture of anger, indignation and depression. They always wish that they had dealt with the situation in a

different, more effective or forceful way at the time. The past preoccupies them rather than the present, as if they would like to make every situation perfect and to their advantage.

5) *Capsicum*
These individuals also live in the past, and their personality is a mixture of irritability and depression. Whatever the situation they want to be elsewhere, feel intensely home-sick and long for the familiar. Any new situation is turned into a threat, and they are always very emotional people.

6) *Naja*
An overwhelming torpor and complete collapsing loss of energy accompanies the depressive state — provoking additional anxiety and restlessness because of a sense of being paralyzed. Palpitations are a frequent feature.

7) *Platina*
The personality has a marked tendency to feelings of superiority, pride and even arrogance which makes them vulnerable, because it is often a defence against feelings of failure and inadequacy. Because of these character traits, hurt pride and rejection is inevitable, and adds to the depression and indignation. Such personalities also live in the past, dwelling on past glories, but they are rarely very effective in the present.

8) *Sepia*
This form of depression gets worse as the day drags on and fatigue and irritability builds up. Irritability directed at those nearest and dearest makes them feel hopeless, worn out and defeated, which is soon transmitted to anyone around. Their pains, constipation and fatigue are all of a 'dragging down' nature. A sadistic punishing element is never far from the surface. Whatever is done or suggested usually ends in failure and irritability.

9) *Phosphoric acid*
This remedy is indicated for more silent, chronic depression with withdrawal. It resembles *Arsenicum,* but these types lack the extreme agitation associated with that remedy. The major preoccupation is with worries for the future, which are not easily reassured.

10) *Nitric Acid*

There is an anxious depression, with irritability, and hypersensitivity to the least trifle — noise, draught, and especially being touched. There is nearly always a chronic, recurrent, painful problem with one of the orifices of the body, which adds to the misery and irritability.

Puerperal Depression

Because of the profound psychological and hormonal changes that occur, and because the mother is especially vulnerable, when depression occurs after childbirth the root causes are often obscure. In some cases the birth has not been well accepted or established as a natural process. Pregnancy may have been unpleasant with constant morning sickness and nausea during the early months and followed by discomfort and malaise later. For some, the pregnancy was unconsciously unwanted, resented and rejected as if a foreign body rather than a culmination of femininity and maternal needs. Sometimes the depression fails to heal naturally and after severeal weeks becomes more disturbing and bizarre, leading to a break with reality and the development of a delusional psychotic illness marked by feelings of persecution and hallucinations. Quite often there have been no warning signs of a severe break-down, with either eccentricity or any tendency to withdraw.

Sometimes the baby itself is rejected, felt to be ugly and is unloved, not a part of the mother — particularly in the early days before the maternal instincts are fully established; (usually this is much more common in the father — where paternal instincts are often slow to emerge.) In severe cases there may be either violent phantasies or actual physical assaults on the baby with battering as an expression of underlying feelings of failure, despair, depression and irritability.

When the baby is felt to be unwanted, such feelings cause severe guilt and depression, especially when the young mother compares herself with others. There is a feeling of being unloving and basically a bad person, failing as a wife and a mother and this is worse whenever there are any feelings of ambivalence.

Depression may follow a traumatic childbirth, particularly when there has been a long and exhausting period of labour, a difficult presentation and delivery which needs to be adjusted and turned. In some cases the head fails to engage properly or the neck of the uterus fails to dilate fully so that forceps and an anaesthetic are required. For others, the depression has been triggered by a caesarian delivery because the health of the mother or child is in danger — this is felt to interfere with the natural process, and there may be sensitivity and vomiting as a reaction to the anaesthetic and psychological situation, which does not heal.

CASE NOTE

A woman of 35 came with a first attack of severe depression since the birth of her first baby some weeks before. Prior to this she had been well and of good personality with no previous periods of depression and always a happy and cheerful person. There were no problems until the immediate labour and birth when the baby presented abnormally — by the face — towards the birth canal. The labour began to be long and drawn out leading to foetal distress and tachycardia — or rapid heart rate of the baby. Because of this and the abnormal presentation, it was neccessary to use forceps to effect the delivery. The mother haemorrhaged after the birth and also required stitching because of the forceps.

Following the birth, the mother was kept in a side observation room for five hours, separated from the baby while blood was matched for a transfusion. She was not told the reason for the long delay, nor could she understand what had happened or get any adequate information. She decided that there must be 'something wrong with her or the baby' as all the other mothers had returned to the ward quickly and she alone found herself isolated in a small observation room, unable to pass water, surrounded by a stream of nurses who kept taking her pulse and blood pressure, but no one gave her any explanations. Although her husband was also present at the delivery and afterwards, this did nothing to relieve the severe anxiety and confusion of the moment, nor relieve the subsequent state of depression. In this case, the depression was brought about by the prolonged period of physical weakness and the lack of information to correct her phantasies or deepest fears.

Recommended Remedies for Puerperal Depression

1) *Sepia*

Especially useful when the condition followed a difficult confinement with severe haemorrhage. Indifference with delusional thinking is marked and such depression may be closely connected with destructive phantasies towards the child. Generally, everything and everyone irritates and is exhausting. Any attempts to reason with or contradict the mother worsens the mental state. Criticism is always a feature — the food, the nursing staff, the doctors or the treatment is wrong, and the patient is the victim or martyr, dragged down to the point of exhaustion by life's tribulations. Always use in the 200c potency.

2) *Platina*

There is a combination of the typical pride and arrogance which is the hall-mark of this personality, with anger, indignation and often paranoia. Instead of the usual excessive pride in the child, paradoxically this is replaced by overwhelming aggressive impulses which provoke the most severe depression and confusional state. Use the 200c potency.

3) *Natrum mur.*
The depression where this remedy is indicated is somewhat different, provoked by an inability to be able to feel and respond with any sense of 'occasion' or joy at the new arrival. Maternal feelings seem minimal and everything is carried out in an automatic fashion, leading to tears, feelings of failure and panic. Generally the problem and the depression is short-lasting, but during the acute phase there is usually a tendency to isolation and to brood. Use the high potencies.

4) *Arnica*
Sometimes a confinement has been unduly prolonged, or a surgical or mechanical (forceps) intervention was required. Use after a delivery when there has been a haemorrhage or shock of any degree. Such depressions are due to a combination of the physical weakness and an emotional reaction to it. They are usually short-lasting. Use the 200c potency.

5) *Aconitum*
This remedy is indicated when the trigger to depression was acute fear during the birth — perhaps the fear that there was 'something wrong' with the baby. The resulting depression may be severe or mild, according to the underlying personality. Use the high 200c potency.

6) *Ignatia*
This remedy is the one of choice whenever, at the time of the confinement, there has also been a severe shock and loss. A close member of the family may have died or been killed in an accident. The infant may have been still-born, or one of a set of twins may not have survived. In all cases severe depression, often with delusional features, has occurred because the personality cannot cope with the loss at such a time of natural vulnerability. Dramatic hysterical features may also occur when the illness has not attained a delusional level with a break with reality. Use the 200c potency.

7) *Staphisagria*
In some personalities, depression occurs after a long, drawn-out, painful and exhausting birth. Often there have been difficulties with the

presentation of the child, or the pelvis, so that a forceps intervention may have been necessary. In general, there are powerful feelings of resentment at having been 'cut about', and always a sense of indignation, leading inevitably to depression, and in some cases rejection of the child, with a more disturbed confusional break-down. In prescribing, use the 200c potency when the mental symptoms are severe. If less severe and mainly of resentment, use the 30c potency thrice weekly.

8) Cimicifuga (Actaea)

There is a severe mental break-down, of unknown cause, with excitement, delusion and confusion leading to puerperal mania, followed by bouts of depression. In many cases the confinement was a difficult one, and the cause of the psychosis may last over many weeks. Use the 200c potency.

Agitated Depression

This is one of the most distressing forms of depression, usually seen in the elderly although it can also occur in the younger age groups when tensions mount and anxiety and fear become intolerable, only finding an outlet by heightened body tone and tension. The whole body shakes with a fine tremor or there may be a coarse, irregular movement of the hands and limbs which causes distress, and is usually worsened in company or in any stress situation. Depression is often severe and near to becoming suicidal at times. Usually, whatever remedies have been taken have either failed or made matters worse. Pessimistic in the extreme, even well indicated homoeopathic remedies or the more powerful nosodes and miasmic remedies fail to evoke any positive response. Like manic-depression, a closely related disorder, this is one of the most difficult syndromes for the homoeopath to resolve satisfactorily. There is an obsessional quality about such depressions so that everything is rigidly seen in the negative, nothing works or is enjoyed and everything is complained about.

The bowels are invariably constipated and a source of severe hypochondriacal preoccupation; often the limbs ache from rheumatism and tension, causing generalized body pains which are a source of anxiety. There is also a lack of interest in food which contributes to the constipation and weakness complained of.

Week by week the individual feels worse, weaker, more depressed, hopeless and defeated by his illness. Equally, they defeat the doctor, every treatment and every therapeutic endeavour. Sepia seems perfectly indicated as a remedy, but they rarely respond. Baryta carb. also does little to relieve the situation. These personalities have the chilliness and obsessional make-up of *Arsenicum*, but this remedy is usually given without any really positive response; similarly with *Zinc met.*, which is associated with all the agitation and depression of the condition. *Sulphur, Medorrhinum, Aurum met.*, all or any of which would seem to be likely remedies to turn the tide of agitation and masochism, usually fail in their turn.

Any improvement, if at all, comes only after several weeks of regular visits and treatments — often when all hope has been given up. Such patients, whatever their response, need a great deal of support and patient caring, yet they can be very exhausting to treat, particularly during the waiting period before there is a response. It is important to carefully and thoroughly check every physical symptom complained of, in order to reassure them and to exclude the possibility of an underlying organic illness. The diet and level of exercise must be adjusted to an optimum for their age. Many are heavily drugged by aperients, sedatives and tranquillizers or anti-depressants, which often serve to aggravate the underlying problem. In addition, they frequently consume large quantities of tea, coffee and cigarettes, and are heavily dependent upon them, in an attempt to find some relief or pleasure in life. Yet such dietary excesses only worsen and aggravate the tension.

There is almost invariably a long-suffering, saintly partner, who is never far away — usually in a martyr-masochistic relationship, giving the clue to the level of unconscious dynamics, and such a relationship has usually been present in this form for many years. Not infrequently, the whole illness and marriage rest upon a chronic sado-masochistic partnership, which is part of the reason why cure and resolution of the problem is often so drawn out, or disappointing.

Often it is only when the doctor finally admits defeat, yet still goes on seeing the patient, when all hope of cure has finally been given up and the patient is seen as incurable, only then does some improvement occur. The patient may have often threatened suicide if the doctor fails or stops the visits and treatment — in spite of its short-comings; the doctor represents a last hope, so that when the patient and the doctor have reached the extremes of defeat, exasperation and hopelessness, then suddenly, for no apparent reason, other than the need to take everything to the extreme — suddenly the patient feels better, smiles again, and gains confidence; the pains ease off. Suddenly there is a response to the indicated remedy — but not before the doctor has been through hell, and after many months of suffering.

Recommended Remedies for Agitated Depression

1) *Arsenicum*

A basic and excellent remedy, but the personality must 'fit'. The basic make-up is chilly, exhausted, fastidious, quite unable to ever relax. Such types worry endlessly about trifles and are obsessional in an attempt to delay all action. Hypochondriasis is marked, and all symptoms are worse after midnight. They are always preoccupied with and fearful of something or other to cause worry and agitation. Use the high 200c potency.

2) *Zinc met.*

The excessive sensitivity of these types provokes the combination of weakness and nervous fidgeting and agitation, especially of the legs and feet, which are never still. The basic personality is withdrawn, silent, depressed and worried. For this condition, only use the 200c potency.

3) *Natrum mur.*

Agitation occurs because of the presence and attempts to help and to be sympathetic made by others, and the least outside approach or offer to assist causes outbursts of anger, followed by increased depression. They want to suffer alone, yet there is agitation as long as they are left to their misery without interference. Use the highest potencies.

4) *Belladonna*

This is indicated for a sudden acute attack of agitation, often violent and unexpected; the face becomes flushed hot and red, the mind confused. Use the 200c potency.

5) *Rhus tox.*

There is a mixture of restless agitation and weeping, so that these patients are quite unable to stay still, and pace or walk up and down. They are often worse in the evening, or for any form of damp or cold. Movement seems essential because of the mental over-activity and standing still in one place is impossible. Painful joints and rheumatism may also be complained of. Use the high 200c potency.

6) *Magnesia carb.*

There is a combination of agitation, depression and tension together with marked exhaustion, cramps and pains which are generalized and seem constant. Constipation and extreme loss of weight are often present. Use in high potency.

7) *Naja*

There is agitated depression with marked exhaustion, palpitations, and frequent left-sided joint or abdominal pains, worse for damp or cold.

8) *Nitric acid*

There is a combination of agitation, weakness and depression, with sharp, typical, splinter-like pains. There is usually a chronic problem in one of the orifices — anal fissure, cracks in the corners of the mouth, or ulceration and soreness in the vulval region — the pains always sudden, lancing and disturbing, which just as quickly go. General twitching is a feature of this nervousness and depression, which is often of a chronic nature. Use the 200c potency.

Psychotic Depression

This is a particularly disturbed and unpredictable state — difficult for both patient and family, as both seem to be talking and thinking at cross-purposes. It differs from depression related to pregnancy or childbirth. Although the onset of the depression may have been slow and imperceptible, the depressive state itself is often sudden and violent, leading at times to a seemingly paradoxical and inexplicable suicide attempt. Such attempts may occur without warning and sometimes after an apparently 'good' period. The commonest age for such problems to suddenly occur is the young adult or, at times, in the 30 to 40 year range.

CASE NOTE

A young university student of 24 had been in hospital for several months with a bizarre depressive disorder, following the break-down of his studies. There had been several previous suicide attempts, but in recent weeks he seemed to be much improved and in a more positive state of mind. He was allowed home for weekend leave, seemed relaxed and happy, talked well with the parents — who had consistently given him a great deal of time and concerned attention — chatted with friends and discussed plans for the future. He seemed content and pleased with his treatment and progress generally, quite happy for the parents to leave him alone for a short time during the afternoon.

During their brief absence, he threw himself from an upper window, killing himself. There had been no clue whatsoever to this violent state of mind, no hints of being suicidal or desperate in any way. During the morning he had been pleasant, relaxed and at ease.

This tragic case clearly demonstrates the degree of 'splitting off' denial and covering up that can occur in a determined psychotic depression. Depression is often covered up in a most plausible way, as part of the often determined attempt to destroy the self — in some other cases, often in a determined final drive to 'foil the enemy'.

There is always a break with reality, meaning a break with both external reality, people and relationships, as well as the more serious break with inner reality — perceptions, judgements and interpretation of people, their messages, intentions and motivations. The break with the inner, stabilizing, psychic reality is unfortunately not always clear to the family for sometimes several months. Often, for years the patient has had many vague, peripheral, esoteric interests — either in such areas as mysticism, religion or philosophy, and the dividing line between an intellectual, metaphysical level of interest and a delusional state is often a fine one until there are more gross manifestations — when the patient hallucinates — and this may be denied or hidden for many months. There is commonly a facade put up to the world — to those others who are against them or unable to understand the importance of their experiences. It is quite common for them to feel that others are plotting against them in some way — often the parents, with their suggestion of treatment. When there is a determined suicidal intention, which the psychotic does not usually see as such, the patient is usually determined not to give the show away, and as it is part of the delusional process, it is kept secret from everyone.

Because of the internal break or fragmentation of the ego, a new, inner delusional reality develops along with a new energy process which does not conform to the 'norm' or reality relationships and expectations as we know them.

The inner psychic world still exists but becomes distorted and built-up of flimsy and fragile assumptions, mis-interpretations and wrong percepts of external reality. Responses eventually become exaggerated and inappropriate, an exaggeration of the previous personality which was, in most cases, either withdrawn or aggressive and rebellious. During the less acute phases psychotics may be shy, unsure of themselves, rather remote and difficult to relate to because of an indefinable, bizarre and disjointed quality to their thought processes. There is a common preoccupation with the opposite sex and with masturbation — but always with a peculiar connotation of guilt. Any artistic or creative attempts seem to be rendered flat or compulsive and inharmonious by the psychotic process, with a tendency for part-objects to emerge — both in speech, ideas and thoughts.

Recommended Remedies for Psychotic Depression

1) *Stramonium*
There is a break with reality, leading to violent and sudden mood changes with swings from severe maniacal excitement to bouts of depression and periods of hallucination. The 200c potency is needed.

2) *Hyoscyamus*
There is the most intense and violent excitability with fear, delusion and delirium, difficult to control. They are overtaken by delusional convictions and visual hallucinations, fearful and suspicious, especially fearing water. A marked diagnostic feature is the intolerance of any form of covering. Depression is never far from the manic stage, and may be inappropriate to the point of obscenity. Always use the highest potencies.

3) *Belladonna*
This is another remedy for manic-depressive activity with delusions and sudden, violent outbursts, followed by equally profound depression. Burning heat and redness is present in the manic stage. Use the 200c potency.

4) *Tarantula hisp.*
There is. the most violent and destructive behaviour, followed by depression, changeable mood, and fear of being alone. Delusional conviction and hallucination is present. Such cases are often very sensitive to music and dancing (*Sepia*), which ameliorates the mood of self-destructive activity. Use in the 200c potency.

5) *Sulphur*
They are less agitated, but in a delusional world of unreality, convinced that the most banal is superlative. Untidy in every aspect, their perceptions and thought processes are equally in disorder and illogical. Burning pains are often present together with a chronic 'dirty-looking' skin complaint. Intolerance of water is frequently a feature. Use in high potency.

6) *Lachesis*
This remedy is indicated for the much more paranoid, suspicious, jealous psychotic depressive — solitary, withdrawn, and full of delusional ideas about others who supposedly betray them, so that finally no one is felt to be trustworthy. Severe depression and

hopelessness is always a feature. Use in the 200c potency.

Suicidal Depression

In any form of depression, whenever there is an overwhelming sense of hopelessness and despair, suicide is always a real risk. The origins are very varied and different, sometimes apparently quite trivial, but basically there is a change from a listless, apathetic state to a more aggressive and actively destructive determination to this time 'do' something — which is nearly always directed at the self. Basically there is a determined desire to terminate life — the exception being the hysterical attempt aimed at drawing attention to pain and suffering and often containing a manipulative element.

True suicidal depression may occur at any age from adolescence onwards. It is rare in childhood, but can even occur during the pre-teenage years in some severe cases. In general, it is most common in late adolescence, with a particularly high incidence in university students where pressures of work and frequently tutor and parental expectations create impossible problems for the student with depressive tendencies. There is often a rigid personality with a marked sense of guilt, where success and ambition are high priority needs. There are commonly feelings of resentment towards the parents; in others, there are problems of jealousy towards another sibling, felt to be more gifted and favoured and under less pressure generally.

When suicidal depression occurs in the young adult, or in an older person, there has commonly been a break-down at an earlier period of life — frequently in early adolscence. This may have been a mild depression or, in some cases, already quite severe. In the suicidal state there is a recurrence of a similar problem, unresolved at the earlier period, which now recurs, more severely this time. A suicidal attempt may occur in marriage when there has been a severe break-down of communications, or when one of the partners is especially vulnerable, for many reasons, and too easily threatened by an outburst of anger, misunderstanding or a period of lack of affection. In such cases, a period of marital difficulty or crisis is built up into a hopeless, impossible situation which can never be resolved.

Of course, the decision to make a suicidal attempt is itself a form of anger and violence, a response to the situation which is turned in upon the self, rather than directed and expressed more openly. In less dramatic cases, the lack of communication is more severe and long-standing, with alienation and isolation, giving way to a sense of failure and desperate hopelessness. Often the person wrongly feels trapped and caught up in a dependent relationship, with no possibility emotionally or financially of becoming independent. In other cases the marriage has been a mistake from the start, and the suicidal attempt is an expression of long-term resentment at being caught up in a disastrous situation which may have occurred originally for neurotic reasons rather than having any base in real love or sharing.

In middle age, severe suicidal depressive impulses may occur as a feature of the 40-year life crisis, often when there are added pressures of a marital crisis, or when loneliness and isolation in a widow or single person reaches intolerable levels. When such impulses occur in the elderly it may reflect the seriousness of a senile delusional illness, or in others a calculated, intellectual decision to terminate life at a certain age, before senility or dependence and physical disability occur. By mutual agreement, such an act may involve both partners, and because it is well planned, sometimes over a period of years, it is successful and the underlying depression is never admitted or comes to the surface.

Suicidal impulses may occur after loss, as part of the mourning process and grief — either immediately or several weeks later. In such cases, there has been a failure of the normal mourning which usually prevents such a tragedy from occuring. A similar state of mind may occur during a chronic, seemingly incurable illness, when there may be a determined, sometimes successful suicidal attempt, but in general this is not common, and feelings of peace and serenity are often more frequent than severe problems of depression.

Recommended Remedies for Suicidal Depression

1) *Aurum met.*
This remedy is indicated for severe states of melancholia, which cannot be lifted by contact or reassurance. There is an overwhelming desire to terminate life and suffering by suicide. Cardiac symptoms are frequently present — especially either as palpitations or angina — and this aggravates the severity of the melancholia. Use in the 200c potency.

2) *Natrum sulph.*
The depression is always worst in the mornings, with silent withdrawal into hopelessness, despair and determined suicidal impulses. There is nearly always an associated respiratory weakness present in addition, which helps to pin-point the correct remedy; there is often chronic bronchitis, or shortness of breath and weakness to aggravate the depression. Use the 200c potency.

3) *Nux vomica*

An irritable, restless melancholia is present with spasmodic but violent impulses to suicide, causing anxiety and fear. The intestinal tract is often involved as a result of the underlying tensions and anxiety, leading to indigestion, constipation or duodenal ulcer. Use the highest potency.

4) *Argentum nit.*

The suicidal problem here is much one of an obsessional compulsive impulse particularly to throw themselves from a window, or feeling 'drawn' by water so that there are suicidal impulses when crossing a bridge. Such impulses are not usually acted upon, but they rather reinforce the obsessional formulaes — the panic and anxiety. Heat in any form is intolerable. Use in the 200c potency.

5) *Alumina*

A mixed depression is present, with impatience and uncertainty. Everything is held back, including the bowel movements, and there is the most severe constipation. There are obsessional fears about anything that could be used as an instrument of suicide. An itchy skin is often present. All aluminium cooking utensils must be changed. Use in the 200c potency.

6) *China*

A severely agitated depressed state is present with exhaustion, often following a long illness or nursing care of a relative. Use the highest potency.

7) *Veratrum alb.*

There is a severe, silent, mute, withdrawn state with determined, often undisclosed suicidal intentions.

Hysterical Depression

This is often a chronic problem with a history of various short-lived bouts of depression, sometimes with several unsuccessful and dramatic suicidal gestures, but no really determined and serious attempts. The underlying problems may have been present in one form or other since childhood and adolescence, with a tendency towards a culmination of pressures to emerge in a dramatic way. Such dramas may have been a feature of the personality make-up for as long as anyone in the near family can recall. In many ways, it is a dangerous depression because such attempts can 'go wrong' — either by error or carelessness turning into tragedy. Yet they are never true attempts to terminate life because the hysteric is far too attached to life and to himself. When an attempt occurs it is always both a protest and a desperate appeal for attention because of the seemingly insoluble problem that dominates them for the moment, and their innter state of anguish and unhappiness. Feelings of frustration and lack of fulfilment are common, whether they are going through a phase of depression or not, and narcissism is always a marked feature.

In many ways attractive people, the hysterical personality tends nevertheless to lack depth and real commitment. They are life's butterflies, intensely involved for a while, then losing interest, quickly bored with others and depressed again, always needing and seeking some new stimulus. Because they cannot forget themselves or their own problems for more than the briefest time, such personalities have great difficulty in being alone because really they are unable to tolerate themselves — disliking their own self-image and what it stands for, in spite of their profound narcissism which does not prevent chronic self-criticism.

These types are frequently on the telephone for lengthy periods in long, animated conversations, falling flat as soon as they replace the receiver. People tend to be collected and wooed to avoid the problem of being alone with themselves and to reassure them that they are lovable, a success, popular and wanted — mainly because they find their own company so boring and intolerable.

The reason for this paradoxical self-dislike when there is so much narcissism, is because of the inability to give out any real love or caring in any depth, or to give of themselves; this is the root cause of many of their problems. Whatever interest, enthusiasm or caring that is developed is nearly always self-directed or contrived and manipulated and therefore narcissistic and part of the absorption with their own problems, physical appearance or difficulties.

In addition there is an excessive attachment and preoccupation with infantile family links, nearly always with one of the parents. There is a tendency to talk endlessly about their grievances in the family — how misunderstood they are by a sibling or parent. Yet at the same time they are quite unable to separate themselves from the personalities involved and complained about. In reality, they seem to be on surprisingly good terms with the persons involved in spite of the complaints. In general, they are quite unable to live their lives or develop to the full as people in their own right because of these excessive ambivalent attachments. They may spend their whole lives talking endlessly about the family and how misunderstood, unappreciated and unloved they are, oblivious to the feelings and needs of those around them.

Because of these excessive infantile and oedipal attachments, a great deal of their adult sexuality is tied up and unavailable, so that they are unable to devote themselves in either a sexual or emotional way, and inevitably feel deprived because of it. Depression eventually and inevitably occurs because they feel they have failed — are unable to love or to be loved. Love is one of the things that matters most of all to them. It is often conceived and desired in very infantile terms — hence it seems so unattainable. This love is what most preoccupies and yet eludes them.

When depressed, the hysterical personality feels desperate for love, understanding and reassurance — really also wanting to recapture an infantile closeness to the mother. The suicidal gesture is often a vain attempt to try and recover what they need most in life and yet are quite unable to give out. The situation often remains a chronic one because there is typically little insight into their own narcissism and it is difficult to overcome other than in exceptional circumstances.

The hysterical personality is never really available as a total person, always seeming remote, lacking interest in the present and too preoccupied with the past or the future. Both the past and the future stimulate them, but the present really leaves them cold because they ultimately lack the confidence to be themselves.

However much attention and reassurance is given however, it is never enough to satisfy or to resolve their problems except for a very short time.

Recommended Remedies for Hysterical Depression

1) *Ignatia*
The person is typically of dark complexion with a changeable dramatic make-up. These personalities commonly explain of a lump in the throat that cannot be explained in any physical terms and is purely due to tension. Many symptoms are odd and seemingly contradictory — the throat pains, for instance, are relieved by food and swallowing. They are always better for music, and there is commonly an unresolved mourning process which is at the root of their problem. Use the 200c potency.

2) *Pulsatilla*
The make-up is nearly always fair, changeable and with a tendency to weep at the least thing. Passive, manipulative and dramatic, their mood is always changeable — from depression to one of laughter and tears.

Any form of heat is intolerable, and worsens their mood. Use in the 200c potency.

3) Cimicifuja racemosa

The behaviour is always extreme with sudden unpredictable bouts of hysterical depression, often associated with rheumatic problems and painful menstruation. Use in the high potencies.

4). Asafoetida

The depression is marked by symptoms of collapse and fainting, a lump in the throat and many intestinal problems of belching, foul gases, distention, a foul taste in the mouth or offensive diarrhoea. Use the 200c potency.

5) Moschus

This remedy is associated with the typical adolescent teenage girl's depression — irritable, uncontrolled giggling, one cheek cold, the other hot. They are often preoccupied with a fear of death and dying. Use the 200c potency.

6) Valerian

The personality is full of fears, imaginations and phantasies — sees the shape of men or animals in the dark. All symptoms are worse in the evening and at night. There is a tendency to be changeable, experiencing twitching, palpitations, loss of identity, confusion and depression. Rheumatic pains are common. Use in the 30c potency thrice weekly.

Depression Following Acute Infections

Depression is common after any long, drawn out, debilitating illness which depletes and drains the body's energies and reserves. Such feelings may follow any minor infection from a severe prolonged common cold; it is also common in cases of more chronic sinusitis or recurrent sore throat, and especially following an attack of 'flu'. Most cases, however, occur during the period of prolonged convalescence from any of the viral epidemic illnesses, particularly hepatitis, glandular fever or influenza.

Depression is also common following acute viral broncho-pneumonia in the young adult when a healthy young person is suddenly laid low for several weeks with a severe bronchial infection which fails to respond to any of the usual and conventional forms of treatment. It is also frequent after shingles — particularly during the period of neuralgia which commonly follows the acute problem of vesicles, with pain due to scarring during the healing phase. This irritates peripheral nerves, causing not only chronic seemingly incurable burning pains, but also the most profound depression. Often the patient feels himself to be in the total grip of the illness and psychologically defeated — still in pain or exhausted after many long weeks of this acute illness.

A similar depressive problem may occur when any of the infective conditions usually seen in the child occur acutely in adult years. The course and progress of such an illness — mumps or chicken pox in the adult — is often severe, painful and long, commonly causing depression because of the severity of the symptoms and the apparent inability of the body to throw off what is felt to be a banal illness.

During the convalescent period from any of the above infections, concentration is difficult, indigestion interfered with, the appetite poor, bowel movements irregular and constipated when there is not a problem of chronic diarrhoea. The level of libido is nearly always depressed which worsens feelings of irritability and defeat. Such depressive problems usually occur only for the period of the physical symptoms, lifting when the underlying condition improves. When recovery is drawn out and slow, the psychological state of depression seems equally hopeless and unending.

Recommended Remedies for Depression Following Infection

1) *The Constitutional Remedy of the Individual*
In order to mobilize energy reserves and a more positive response, give this remedy in the 200c potency, and repeat in 6-8 weeks if the response is still weak.

2) *Give the Nosode of the Specific Illness*
I recommend that this be given at an early stage in the treatment in the 30c potency thrice weekly for a month. Some of the most frequently used nosodes are *Influenzinum* and the *Hepatitis* nosode; the *Glandular fever* nosode is of especial value in what is often a long drawn out and depressing illness. *Morbillinum* (measles nosode) and *Varicella* (chicken pox nosode) are also available.

3) *China*
For problems of depressing weakness and exhaustion, loss of appetite and energy reserves. Insomnia is common and reflects over-activity of the mind, so that in spite of the weakness and tiredness and longing for sleep and rest, they cannot really relax or let the mind be still. Use the 200c potency.

4) *Cadmium phos.*
For the depressive problems after a long drawn out viral illness such as Influenza, when the patient seems unable to rally from the exhaustion and lacks all forms of vital response and fight. Use the 30c potency thrice weekly.

5) *Arnica*
This remedy in the low 6c potency is often of help during the slow and difficult climb back from a long and depressing convalescence after an acute illness.

Menopausal Depression
Cessation and lack of regularity in the monthly flow is one of the most difficult periods of psychological adjustment in a woman's life. It is a time of great uncertainty and unpredictability for most women as the menstrual cycle either stops completely or becomes either intermittent or excessive. This lack of normal hormonal rhythm often fills the woman with overwhelming feelings of emotional uncertainty. Not only may flooding be a worrying and disturbing aspect of the period, but there may also be floods of tears and emotion, sometimes of drenching night sweats with flashes of sudden heat. All of this creates not only physical discomfort, but also anxiety and a sense of weakness and uncertainty. This weakness may be physiological in origin when there is exhaustion from severe anaemia due to the heavy loss, but it may equally have a psychological basis because of underlying depression and the changes that have to be adapted to.

Some women are more fortunate and the 'change' passes as a non-event, almost unnoticed; suddenly a period is missed, does not recur for several months and then quietly disappears with no adverse reactions. For many it is a time of anxiety, panic and depression — a time of emotion and tears with fear of break-down. Affairs are common, often fleeting and unsatisfactory, leading to an increased sense of futility and defeat. An adolescent re-emergence of preoccupation with the body image may occur, so that slimming becomes an obsession and staying beautiful becomes the centre point of life — part of the need for reassurance against fears of ageing and ultimately death. When there is a preoccupation with weight-loss, there is often also an unending fight against the need to indulge in sweet fattening foods as a compensation for feelings of being unloved and unnoticed — really unloving and unnoticing. Such needs and cravings for attention and for love are much the same as in teenage years, with a similar re-emergence of narcissism and less concern for the needs of others which is one of the major root-causes of the depression.

Coupled with the narcissistic tendencies and self-centredness is an increasing dislike and criticism and even hate of the self, especially of the physical appearance, which can enter into the depressive image of the self. When severe, such self-destructive masochistic attitudes can completely destroy all self-confidence, creating an added need for reassurance from others. All of this creates a vicious circle — as the dislike of self and self-criticism increases, so too the dietary cravings are indulged, often in sudden bouts of 'breaking out'; this can lead to all the adolescent problems of skin blemishes, or adolescent acne, together with obesity from fluid retention. Such problems add to the gynaecological and menopausal complications and uncertainties and to the state of psychological unrest, uncertainty, loneliness and depression.

Recommended Remedies for Menopausal Depression

1) *Sepia*
The periods are late or delayed with profuse flow, often flooding with black clots. The typical irritability, fatigue, constipation and backache are nearly always present to some degree. Use the 200c potency.

2) *Lilium tig.*
Irritability and anger are frequent, worse for any attempts at consolation (*Natrum mur.*) and made worse by the dragging-down uterine pains. This remedy is linked with always being in a hurry, always restless, and only better for walking in the fresh air. Give the 200c potency.

3) *Iodum*
There is a nervous and restless state of depression, with variable and unreliable periods, so that the woman never knows where she is with her dates. The remedy is associated with warm-bloodedness, flashes of heat, and relief only in a cool atmosphere. Use the 30c potency thrice weekly for a month.

4) *Pulsatilla*
The woman is depressed, emotional and tearful. The flow is weak or absent, sometimes dark with clots, but always variable and unreliable. Use the 200c potency.

5) *Thuja*
The periods are excessive, dark with clots and painful. A low, left-sided ovarian pain is a common problem and occurs during the flow. In general, the woman is depressed, agitated and unable to properly relax.

Sometimes there are bizarre ideas. Use in the 30c potency thrice weekly.

6) *Causticum*
There is a moderate depression, the periods are late and, when present, occur during the daytime only.

7) *Cactus*
The depression is one of silence and withdrawal, becoming irritable if any demands are made or with attention. The periods occur too soon, the flow thick and black, but stopping as soon as the woman lies down. Usually some evidence of cardiac weakness is also present — either as frank angina or as palpitations, which heightens anxiety. Use the high 200c potencies.

Depression in the 40-Year-Old
This is largely a male problem, but not entirely. Similar problems occur in the woman, but are overshadowed by the more external preoccupations with adjusting to the menopause. For the male, the first disagreeable intimations of mortality occur in the mid-30s and early 40s, as physical and hormonal changes make themselves more obvious. Psychologically, this is always a time for a profound reappraisal of life's aims and goals, accompanied by a sense of loss and a feeling that youth is at an end. In reality it is the end of a psychological era — of seemingly timeless idealization and boundless possibilities to be thought about and mused over for the future. Suddenly time is no longer on one's side and there is a sense that opportunities are fewer. Until this age it seemed that any decisions and commitments could be further delayed because of having youth and time.

Not all, but many women feel that it is too late to have a child at this age and men have an unpleasant sense of being too old at 40. Jobs advertised are aimed at a younger age-group so that work areas, plans and projects for the future have to be looked at in a more realistic way. It may be necessary to accept that some of the plans may never be realized now, and for some there is a sense of bitterness and regret, of time wasted.

Frequently also, there is a feeling of having achieved a material, even an emotional success without having achieved any real wisdom or faith. A quality of depth and spiritual realization is felt to be lacking, a profound reason for it all. Ambitions realized may seem hollow and somehow empty. Perhaps the marriage is one of pretence, an empty shell — often broken abruptly with a determination to return to new standards, aims and a more authentic way of life. This is often too a time of severe depression when everything seems a burden, all achievements irrelevant — this is the depression of success, of conventionality, of the self-made man.

Such a depression is felt to follow inevitably — a sacrifice of ideals and standards to the service of materialism, and ambition and status — the motor car, washing machine, public school, mortgage. It is also felt to be the price paid for irretrievable lost time and a quality of life and ideals once present, but now submerged under a complicated commitment to gadgets and possessions, time and space fillers, of little real appeal or value.

During such a crisis, affairs are common — often with a younger person. These may often be at the expense of a well-established and apparently happy relationship, in an ultimately self-destructive attempt to recapture lost youth, lost opportunities, lost ideals and intentions and lost time for caring and loving. In most cases, such affairs almost inevitably turn sour and prove not to be the idealized opportunity envisaged, adding to the trail of depressions, regrets, guilt, and often ending in either a broken marriage and family, or one that is irreparably hurt and damaged. The occasions and opportunities in the past, the general tendency to look back with hind-sight and regret often serves as a difficult but fundamental barrier to more healthy, creative thinking and caring, which must ultimately occur in order to resolve the underlying fear and depression.

Recommended Remedies for Depression in the 40-Year-Old

1) Nux Vomica
At this age, the typical Nux personality is often depressed, with a tendency to look back to the past with regret at lost opportunities and chances. They also inevitably look back at old scores and resentments with bitterness. The typical picture is always that of the hard-working, perfectionist personality — more successful in business than at home because of their irritability and outbursts. Hypersensitive to an extreme degree, they are intolerant and rarely ever know how to relax; when they do, time seems to pass so slowly that they just have to do something in order to occupy their state of heightened tension. These types often feel that a material success has been achieved at the expense of their own development. They feel inadequate, are unhappy, irritable and unsatisfied.

2) *Arsenicum*
At 40 the typical obsessional, driving personality is at a peak of rigid, confined thinking, always looking back with regret and forward with fear. These individuals already look and feel old and worn, unable to mobilize any 'animal' warmth so that they are cold on the warmest day. The mind, like the body, is never at rest, constantly agitated, lacking the drive and the courage of the *Nux vomica* types and the ability to make changes. Such a person feels locked into a relentless pattern of routine and humdrum, from which he cannot escape. The often chronic chest problems add to the feeling of weakness and ill health. He is still a 'natty dresser' — but to what avail or satisfaction! Use the 200c potency.

3) *Lycopodium*
At this age the sensitive, unsure personality feels that life is past, and as his energy reserves lessen, he becomes increasingly introspective and hypochondriacal. He is still full of ambitious ideas for the future but these will never be realized. Little confidence has ever really been gained, just a way of coping with life's limitations and avoiding any real confrontation, or dialogue with others. The physical needs of the body at this age are neglected and he tends to enter into a premature decline — still making fine promises, though nobody believes him any longer, least of all himself.

4) *Natrum mur.*
At the age of 40, these types are chronically depressed and lonely, isolated by choice even within a relationship, and still eschewing all real contact with others. He has no sense of drive or direction, is tired and can see no goals for the future, or little satisfaction from the past. He remains as rigid as ever in many of his opinions and attitudes and seems not to have moved with the times.

Mourning and Grief Reactions
Mourning is the normal psychological reaction to loss. Such reactions may last for many months and their absence may be just as abnormal as an excessive reaction, heralding trouble and sickness in the weeks to come. Primarily, mourning is a reaction to separation and loss, ultimately an acknowledgement and recognition of the reality and inevitability of death. Freud considered mourning to be a normal psychological response and part of the essential 'working-through' or emotional acceptance of the loss. He also considered that one aspect of mourning was an unconscious attempt to recreate the dead person. But there are several stages or phases of the mourning response, each of which varies with the individual.

Mourning is a way of coming to terms psychologically with the loss, and during this period of readjustment, and reintegration, particularly after a long and close relationship, this situation has to be restructured in the psyche. Mourning allows a new relationship with the lost person to occur, which at the same time is protective as it prevents life being paralyzed by a prolonged and abnormal period of grief.

The mourning reaction is always more severe when sudden, unexpected and without any psychological warning. When loss is more predicted, it may be thought of as a relief from suffering, particularly in cases of a painful or terminal illness. Loss is inevitably extremely painful to bear when the ties are close, and this can provoke a more severe reaction of pain and grief. When unexpected, as through a violent accident, or involving a child or younger person, death is experienced as a particularly cruel, unjustifiable and senseless blow and the reactions are a form of protestation against fate. Such reactions are frequently violent and masochistic, leading in a few rare cases to actual harm or suicide in some cases. Such violent reactions were considered by Freud to be unconsciously aimed at the lost person — felt to have abandoned them — so that the suffering is partly felt to be their fault, and a punishment or a revenge for not having loved and cared sufficiently.

Such feelings are the cause for the self-reproach that is common in the early days of mourning, when there is a sense of responsibility and guilt for what has happened. Either oneself or others are blamed for the death, with a common feeling that they should have acted sooner, done more to have forseen and prevented it — the feelings of guilt increasing the suffering. When there is an hysterical element to the personality make-up, mourning may become uncontrollable, prolonged and dramatic. It may be dangerous when the person is isolated and unsupported without friends or family to share the burden and often the problems which arise.

The acute phase of mourning lasts for several weeks with insomnia, loss of appetite and fearfulness, especially when alone. Grief reactions may occur following the loss of anyone close, or once close — perhaps in childhood. A much-loved pet who has filled an emotional need over the years causes a form of mourning as with a person, although such reactions are inevitably less severe and prolonged than those involving a member of the family.

But all mourning reactions are painful because of the need for a reintegration of oneself and a coming to terms with one's own mortality and omnipotence. In order to overcome mourning an internal psychological change must occur, accepting the loss, pain and guilt.

Such an acceptance gives a degree of maturity and depth to the personality since mourning involves the depths of the psyche and problems of readjustment in the most profound areas of caring and acceptance of separation and loss. To recognize that even those whom we love the most are not our possessions is a realization which, once accepted, gives a certain depth and maturity.

Sometimes the loss occurs in a situation where the persons have lived in a vacuum or total dependence on the other, and once alone, feel totally lost and hopeless. In such cases, the mourning process may turn into a depressive illness which may culminate in a premeditated suicidal act or in a physical illness, from which the person has no real will or drive to recover, reflecting the severity of the underlying depression.

Recommended Remedies for Mourning and Grief Reactions
Mourning and grief are perfectly normal reactions following loss and it is absolutely essential for the continuation of health that they be allowed to occur without interference other than support and comfort. Help is needed only in those cases where the reaction is abnormal or excessive, or when problems of insomnia or fear and anxiety are overwhelming.

1) *Ignatia*
Because of the basic hysterical make-up, the *Ignatia* patient copes with such loss very badly. The loss seems to provoke an acute fear of death and to increase the lack of confidence already present. The tendency is to become increasingly fearful, like a child fearful of nightmare — indeed earliest fears often come to the surface at this time with the frequent need for a light during the night hours. The least thing throws them into a panic and into a fluctuating melancholia. The dramatic, childish and attention-seeking needs are never far away however. Use the 200c potency.

2) *Natrum mur.*
This is the other major remedy which rivals *Ignatia* for use as the initial prescription. The difference often centres around the needs of *Ignatia* patients for contact with other people, and the abhorrance of such sympathy associated with *Natrum mur. Ignatia* types need others in order to constantly reinforce their own dependent hysterical nature, ensuring people are at their beck and call. *Natrum mur.* individuals are moved to irritability and incensed rage at such manipulations and contact, which feels to them like an intrusion of privacy. Use the 200c potency.

3) *Opium*
There is a mixture of panic and depression after the original acute fear reactions. Constipation to the point of blockages and collapse are the other typical features. Use in the 30c potency.

4) *Gelsemium*
An over-reaction is typical, with extreme nervousness and emotion causing anxiety, fear, panic and depression.

5) *Veratrum alb.*
The reaction is one of absolute shock and defeat by fate and events. These types seem quite unable to take in or cope emotionally with what has happened, sinking into a state of mute withdrawal.

Anniversary Reactions
These are unconscious psychological reactions to an earlier loss and are really mourning reactions in miniature, occurring at the time of year of the original loss. Such reactions occur over a number of years after the original trauma and are marked by a period of flatness and depression. Such anniversary reactions are not recognized by the persons involved, although close members of the family are intuitively often aware of what is occurring. There is typically a period of withdrawal or irritability, sometimes of self-recrimination, and it is common to dream of the lost person — often as a nightmare or fear reaction dream. Such dreaming may occur at the same time of year over a long period and often open the way to a flash of silent remembering. For others, there is a period of compulsive discussion and recall of the past, a looking at old photographs, or talk of what might have been.

Not infrequently it is a time of physical illness with bouts of insomnia and indigestion, sometimes constipation or backache. Others go down with a cold or 'flu' each year regularly and during these anniversary reactions some of the typical mourning features of loss of drive and libido also occur. When a physical illness occurs, it is important for both physician and patient to be able to link the development of symptoms to an unresolved mourning process in order to be able to resolve what is often a chronic recurrent depression. Usually the patient has not recognized the link himself and these seasonal annual lows or illnesses seem quite obscure and without obvious reason. The doctor must combine any treatment with a clear explanation of the underlying psychology.

Often, however, the patient himself gives the clue, provided that the doctor-patient relationship has been given enough time for sensitive listening and for such links and insights to emerge. The homoeopathic relationship, with its balanced emphasis on both the mental as well as the physical disorder, is an ideal approach to allow such links to emerge. Once the link has been understood, symptoms and destructive reactions are usually quickly resolved, and there is a rapid return to confidence and normality.

1) *Natrum mur.*
This oft-recurring remedy in nervous problems is linked with a periodicity that makes for a recurrence of reactions of loss or hurt, coupled with tendencies to repetition and compulsion as one aspect of the obsessional make-up. Because the isolation, shock and grief are deeply locked in, they cannot be naturally 'worked through', and are therefore inevitably buried and repressed, only to surface at other times — often as acutely as the original feelings.

2) *Nux vomica*
Like the elephant, the *Nux* personality never forgets either a slight or a loss which seems almost like a failure and something which should not have occurred — or which they should have been able to control. The symptoms are not those of depression and failure, but may involve the intestines with colic or acute indigestion. Use the 200c potency.

3) *Ignatia*
This is the great remedy for problems of loss and grief which, because of the hysterical elements inevitably present, become deflected into infantile manipulations and a further excuse for dramatic behaviour. This lessens the true feelings of the time, and the ability of the psyche to properly resolve them. Therefore such feelings tend to constantly recur, until the problems of loss, mortality and adjustment are eventually admitted by the psyche. Use the 30c potency thrice weekly until the crisis is passed.

4) *Aconitum*
When fear was the dominating feature at the time of the loss, causing panic and despair, then such reactions and feelings are likely to recur — this is because the fear has never been properly looked at or resolved. Use the 200c potency.

8.

EXISTENTIAL MALAISE

There can be few people that really believe that the ultimate quality of life is purely a materialistic one. For the majority, it must also include the intangibles — the poetry and the mystery of life the spiritual side of man — his beliefs, morals, hopes, wisdom and standards, especially perhaps the ultimates of life, its meaning and shape as well as our role, contribution and destiny within it.

The writings of such contemporary European philosophers as Sartre, Camus, Kierkegaard and equally such varied poetry as that of *The Rubáiyát* and the works of Blake and Housman, have all highlighted the common moral and spiritual crisis which every sensitive human being must face at some time as a consequence of increased sensitivity and awareness, maturity and ageing.

The basic problem is the natural outcome of man's capacity to think. To think intuitively and not just logically is to be aware, to reason, seek and reflect. It is an outcome of man becoming *Homo sapiens*. The questions which inevitably arise at some time are nearly always enigmatic, philosophic and centred around moral doubts; and the answers can be equally perplexing. Such questions reflect extreme personal doubts and private fears and beliefs. Personal anguish of this kind is rarely discussed with anyone — perhaps wrongly — through fear of being thought either a heretic, a fool, just ungrateful or sick-in-the-head. Because of the nature of these underlying philosophic and moral doubts and the intrinsic difficulties in phrasing or defining them, there can be no easy formal answers or direct replies. It is not surprising that the replies and conclusions are as equally imprecise and vague as the questions.

Existential awareness and concern centres around the basic meaning of life, faith, morals, philosophy, man's belief in himself and the meaning and purpose of our stay here. Man has a natural awareness of his transience and ultimate vulnerability and fragility. There is often a deep feeling of aloneness; ultimately of being a very small cog in a very large wheel — a minute particle in a vast whole — rather than of being that whole. At times there is a sense of both nothingness and of everything in terms of the infinite; and none of these feelings or the sense of awareness can in any way be put into satisfactory words by the person or for that matter by the writer.

The above is by way of approach to existential awareness. Existential malaise is the feelings of despair and loneliness, inevitability and acceptance, albeit wary acceptance, that accompanies such awareness, and is an intrinsic part of the uncertainty of the questions, seemingly impossible to resolve.

We live in a society where there is a generalized crisis of beliefs and faith. The most supposedly close-knit religious family often cannot face and discuss death, ageing or dying when faced with it in reality. It was Aristotle who commented that those who know nothing of dying often know nothing either about living and have nothing meaningful to say about it. The present spiritual crisis is every bit as important as any industrial, inflationary, unemployment or monetary crisis, but only gets minimal media coverage. One of the worst features is that people no longer talk about it either — in fact, people don't talk at all. Many have lost faith and interest in almost everything and see no reason why they should do anything other than work and exist for the moment.

In almost every home in Europe or the U.S. families sit night after night, unselectively watching 'rubbish' on the television. Usually they are watching contrived programmes which are of no interest to them; they are glued to the set, not thinking, not talking, passive. Children rush home from school to sit as close as possible to the screen, and any talk centres around the television programmes — when there is any talk at all. In some families, the set is left on when a visitor arrives, the sound is sometimes turned down so that the silent screen can be watched as often as possible and in some cases the sound is not even lowered.

This is the pattern, night after night, week in, week out, and it is not the fault of the television, it is a symptom of our society. People don't read any more either; people don't talk any more and people don't think any more. Doubtless if there wasn't a television, there would be something else invented to take its place, equally mindless and time-filling. A satellite television programme was staged recently with 300 million people watching for a period of two hours. The amount of time lost in total to passive watching is colossal, and most of it is to wipe out personal awareness and the experience of our existential awareness.

In all these examples, the great impulse is in fact to drive out thought and to become unaware. In much the same way as television is a 'time-spinner' of the first order, the drug Valium promotes a conveniently relaxed state of mind. To be able to opt out, take a pill on demand, put on a television programme, have a 'shot', or listen to a record at maximum volume, this is the aim. We have become a nation of extinguishers, mostly self-extinguishers, to the detriment of the quality and the awareness of our lives. The deepest sense and knowledge of this self-extinction is a deep cause for concern and malaise and leads to an increase in existential anxiety for many people.

Faced with such absolute denial and obliteration by the great majority of the inevitable existential challenge, with such radical defences against their admission or even the possibility of their existence, illness both mental and physical is on the increase. It is also highly likely that damage is done to the body by a constant stream of electrons, electron dot-images producing the screen image, and low but continuous X-ray exposures. When will these finally be admitted to as dangers to health and powerful causes of insomnia, over-activity and of behaviour disturbance in the young? It is not surprising that in our society today, one which has become increasingly materialistic, technological and mechanistic, where all too often political expediency is put before people, a lack of faith is commonly expressed. Almost across the board, there is a complete loss of faith in the system — work, politics, politicians and money, religion and the old pillars of the establishment, which once set and represented values and morals worthy of emulation. In nearly all people, whatever their race, creed or class, there is a general feeling that the present society is one of shifting sand, basically unreliable and frequently amoral.

There can be added feelings of loneliness because often there is no inner confidence and all too often no one to externally identify with for support either. This gives an added poignancy to the feeling of being basically on one's own and is a further contribution to the sense of existential malaise.

Loss of faith has become a common problem. It is increasingly widespread and the cause of much pain and suffering, confusion and anguish. In most cases it is the elderly who suffer most of all, and the frequent problem of physical isolation worsens the distress. This existential malaise is not fundamentally a depressive problem, although it may stimulate apparently depressive feelings. The problem is one of man's existence, the meaning and purpose of life, loneliness, direction, faith and belief. These are not easy subjects to grapple with alone, and usually there is no support or understanding within the family situation. Because there are no easy answers, when an attempt is made to discuss and to share the problem, there is often an aggressive response.

The relationship of man to his environment, to God and to his fellow men, are all questions as to the ultimate quality of and reason for life. How and where to live for oneself, for one's family, standards, ideals, values, attitudes, one's role, and the reason for it are all thought about. Naturally there are no quick recipes or immediate easy answers, and for some this may be a cause of anxiety, particularly when the external world and values themselves are so chaotic, confused and changing.

For some, life is much more simple. These people have established beliefs and certainties, or the lack of them. The immediate satisfactions they experience give enough meaning to life and is what counts for them. They have an external goal; outside work, social contacts and external gratifications and pleasures only. Little else seems to matter. They have no time for philosophic questions which seem to have so little relevance and seem ridiculous, at least for the present — and that is what matters. They get on with their jobs, with life, mind their own business and avoid worrying unnecessarily about anything. They may be the fortunate ones but this is doubtful and the price they pay for such indifference is one of depth and awareness.

For others, life remains uncertain and is not so simple, sewn up and straightforward. They are aware of and concerned about the quality of their lives at a deep level; their minds are in a state of flux, but they retain and are in touch with a quality of mystery and of awareness. Their mind and ideas are not fixed, but open, unsure and undogmatic, because they do not know all the answers.

Existential malaise, one aspect of existential awareness, is different from formal anxiety or depression which is commonly seen, although at times it may enter into either, particularly when there are any obsessional or schizoid tendencies to distort reality. In general, the ability to accept a degree of 'not knowing' and uncertainty about life is the culmination of health. In many ways too, nothing is more certain in life than change and death. The ability to be able to tolerate a situation of uncertainty, a problem which cannot be immediately resolved, and to be able to accept a position of anguish is also one of strength. Having the resilience and the strength to bear such doubts without having to immediately 'do' something about them is a test of maturity.

In a problem of emotional illness, the emphasis is always on absolute certainty, on knowing without doubt, on absolute conviction. The deluded, obsessed individual is convinced beyond question, that for instance, without his particular ritualistic precautions, harm will come to him. The depressive is utterly convinced of his unworthiness and that he deserves a fate worse than death. It is very difficult to persuade him to the contrary, whatever the realities. The paranoid personality knows beyond any doubt that there is a plot to discredit and destroy him and that others are against him. When such indefinables are absorbed into or become part of an illness then they become symptoms of an overall mental disturbance to the detriment of the individual who loses any potential for increased awareness or expansion of the mind.

The other manifestation of this overall pattern of denial is the urgent rush and need to be impulsively involved in any new fad, therapy, religion, diet or gadget that the media can most plausibly put over as 'good'. Even the so-called therapies that advocate talking as a 'good, healthy' thing, involving sharing and expression, often miss the point, so that everything is either contrived or artificial and almost invariably too quick or too repressive, sometimes too cathartic, and often ending up as a positive danger to the individual. There is an urgent rush to get away from the self, from awareness, from thinking and knowing, from depth into theory, into the new or back into the old, at all costs, away from a present intuitive awareness and self-knowledge.

All of this is at a cost, often financial, as well as of vital energy and time. Sometimes such flights from knowing and feeling can be at the expense of the family or the marriage or of the children. All too often when the couple should spend more time talking intuitively and sharing their feelings and concerns, the subject is turned off and the 'tele' turned on. At such times, it is frequent to change the subject or plan another spending spree to avoid the listening, the caring and reflection. Naturally such artificial spending, often compulsively as a defence against knowing, is costly to the family budget and serves to create unnecessary inflation and artificial values where nothing is really appreciated or enjoyed for more than the briefest period. Such defences are ultimately harmful to the very fabric of our society because of the artificial demands that they make, and because of the way in which they undermine the depths of sensitivity of the individual and his perceptions.

Man has the underlying wish and the potential to know and to realize himself more fully and completely, provided that he is not dictated to by fears and impulses to obliterate — in the last analysis — the self. Obliteration and denial is not a natural process, however much it may seem to be, and there is a price to pay, often involving emotional health and balance with increased vulnerability to break-down. This is because we become alienated from a natural flexibility when no longer in contact with our deepest selves, however painful that contact may be.

The Nature of Mental Illness

The patient with the typical neurotic anxiety or depressive problem is commonly a paradoxical mixture of uncertainty and overwhelming conviction and certainty. Basically, this type of individual lacks self-confidence and trust, with multiple fears and anxieties of coping, meeting others, including adequacy at work and wherever any demand is made. In all these areas he is typically unsure, full of doubts and wanting to run away from both imagined and real pressures.

But these areas of doubt are usually secondary to such a personality's inner convictions; certainty and confidence are, surprisingly, the major features of his make-up. There is almost invariably a strong and usually total conviction and certitude that in the neurotic areas of attitudes towards others and what is about to happen to them, their own failings or those of others, there are feelings of overwhelming inadequacy. In some ways there is a sense of being trapped by this very certainty, whatever form it takes, and this can be their undoing psychologically because of the problems it creates.

In general, the more mentally ill the person, the stronger the convictions and the certainties. In psychosis, the difference is that the certitudes develop a delusional intensity and a quality that can no longer be differentiated from reality. Such certainty is often felt to have meaning in terms of suffering, punishment, deprivation and supposed malice. Any doubts as to the objectivity of such convictions are accepted with the greatest difficulty and irritation.

Generally in emotional illness there is an intolerance of uncertainty and therefore any doubts are quickly translated into additional concrete, neurotic beliefs. In his depression, the neurotic is just as confident — he knows and is certain as to his beliefs and phobias. In his mind is the certainty that others are wrong when they try to reassure or dissuade him from his feelings of failure, guilt and blame — thus, this very certainty often ensures that treatment is prolonged and difficult. Ask any agoraphobic if he is sure that he can't make it outside. He will inevitably reply with sincerity and conviction that he would almost certainly faint, collapse or have a heart attack if he were to attempt it. Indeed the very thought is often such an ordeal as to bring sweat to the brow.

Existential malaise, as opposed to mental illness, is the awareness of uncertainty. Existential health is the ability to accept this position of uncertainty without having to deny it or to resolve it either. Uncertainty and the pain of not knowing about death, other than its inevitability, is painful and can be a lonely experience. Existential malaise is the direct expression of such anxieties. At the same time, unlike the neurotic position, it does not lead to alienation from others — quite the contrary. Even if such private musings are rarely spoken of, there is usually an added closeness towards and need of others, an understanding, a greater sense of being linked and of interdependence with others, rather than of being in a position of isolation, alienation, despair and manipulation.

Existential doubts are healthy ones rather than doubts based on magical thinking or obsessional certainty or conviction. These are primarily doubts and concerns as to our role and place in the universe. At the same time such natural concerns as to our existence, present in each one of us, only become a significant factor in mental illness when suppressed. Such denial tends to be most marked in adults and the older age groups where the trappings of 'success' and the mechanistic defences of our society are most strong — the emphasis on ease, convenience and gadgetry rather than communication, sharing and inner awareness. It is possible that the roots of mental illness lie at this level in a direct flight from recognition of our existential position. The very deepest meaning of illness becomes an obliteration of mortality by means of an omnipotent illness.

In response to homoeopathic therapy, even in severe emotional problems, there is usually a return to existential awareness and concern without the earlier need for or degree of denial and obliterations, so that human problems can be given more expression and are acknowledged. As this happens, so the patient becomes more of a person again and more human too. It is important that each patient is able to see and to tolerate such doubts and concerns as normal and part of his return to wholeness. The resolution of existential awareness and concern is primarily a matter for each individual to attain; it is not the concern of the physician other than to ensure that there is no confusion with illness or a return to unwarranted treatment.

The problem is a spiritual and a moral one, but the often deep sense of aloneness and sometimes of sadness is not depressive in origin. Uncertainty or doubt about one's role, the meaning and purpose of life is healthy. There is no schizoid break with reality, however, and no move towards withdrawal or isolation, unless the existential problems become a part of a schizoid or obsessional illness with a constant rumination as to the 'meaning of life'.

Often there is a loss of faith and the alienation anxiety is experienced at a spiritual level. There is no formal illness as such, but there are common symptoms of nausea and boredom with life at times, with the frequent sense of loneliness and isolation that is difficult to express or define. Ultimately, man is alone, especially for many of the deepest and most personal areas of spiritual concern and awareness, however many people are in the vicinity.

Homoeopathy helps to broaden and free the mind and allows such philosophic knots to be acknowledged and dealt with more openly and more creatively. The great danger always is of confusing such existential uncertainty with emotional and mental illness, healthy loneliness and solitude with depression, and this is one of the major roles of the physician at all times, as the patient can easily get confused and often requires some guidance in this particular area.

A schizophrenic patient, the acute psychosis burned out, now in his forties, unable to work from lack of experience and confidence, told me, 'I have no soul, it is burned out with my emotions, by my medications and my illness. I have lost my soul, it is separate from my body and it is a cause of infinite sadness for me.' The patient had been undergoing homoeopathic treatment for several months when he came to this realization and depth of communication and awareness.

Another patient, aged 35, made a complete recovery from a long-standing and incapacitating agoraphobic illness. With the improvement, the increase in confidence and ease of travel, came a much greater depth of thought and awareness — at least to the surface. She had no formal training in any area; she needed to 'do' something 'meaningful' and there was a strong feeling of lack of self-fulfillment. She described how she had tried many things in the past — pottery, photography, reading, languages — and none of them gave her a depth of satisfaction. She felt that life was slipping past and was never going to find what she was seeking for. She was very happily married, and there were no material problems; she was attractive, but all the time there was a sense of emptiness, meaningless and searching. She felt her life was taken up with mundane things. She described being sad, but not depressed, always worst at period times when every woman is more in contact with her depths and perhaps her sense of mortality. She feared reaching 50 and being full of regrets — a prospect which frightened her. Many of her friends seemed to feel fulfilled by their children, yet she feared that if she had a family that it might hamper her in her search for more meaning and depth; at the same time she felt guilty about such feelings and that she should have children before it was too late.

During this period of searching, the patient felt at her best when walking in the country, near to birds and animals, or in the garden, growing and caring for her plants. Other 'good' areas were music, reading and quiet for some part of the day, though not in any formal meditation. Exercise, often quietly rather than in a competitive way, was also helpful — swimming, tennis and especially walking. There was a sense that what she was seeking needed to contain all of these positive elements for her — fresh air, good wholesome food, exercise and a feeling of 'at-oneness' with nature. She described feeling like a butterfly, flitting from one creative hobby and interest to another in her search for the indefinable, at the same time feeling guilty that she was not satisfied.

The patient went on further to describe a sense of drifting like a boat without a rudder, never completely involved or in any way permanently taken up with anything, as whatever she undertook seemed to be the wrong thing. 'I feel as if I am seeking intangible things — as if following a fine thread of happiness from which I can be easily thrown off balance.' She then described being scared of sharing such feelings with others in case she might make a fool of herself; she also felt that others didn't have this problem and that she was isolated with it. She was a person who found no solace in the usual social props — smoking, drinking and noise. Finally, she described that while she felt 'better' in herself, able to move around more freely, more complete and 'normal' as a person, this did not dispel her feelings of lack of fulfillment, her search for an identity. All these feelings and awareness were acknowledged for a little while and then squashed back out of sight again until the next time — hence the concern and the existential sadness.

9.

FEARS AND PHOBIAS

It is well known that many people have some form of irrational fear or phobia which, although annoying at times, does not unduly interfere with their lives or healthy functioning. Usually there are no adequate rational explanations that can account for such feelings, the exception being those rare cases of acute fright or trauma — perhaps a fall or near-drowning, causing severe anxiety at the time and now avoided because of phobic feelings.

Often the fear is of something quite small, quick-moving and uncontrollable, particularly when the fear involves small insects or reptiles, especially spiders, mice or snakes. When there has been no trigger-fright situation in earlier years, the fear may have been induced by a parent in infancy who 'passed on' or projected his own fears onto the child — as a way of controlling them, often repeating a process which occured when the parent was in his earliest infancy, and which is beyond recall.

In others, the fear cannot be explained in this way and the threatening situation seems much more to relate to primitive, unconscious anxieties — more in keeping with Freudian theories of dreams and 'part-objects' than conscious realities. Freud described vividly in his early psycho-analytic case material, many examples of unconscious phantasy. These were usually from children but they were also found widely in adults too where, as a result of the inevitable frustrations of life and insatiable baby demands, the parents came to be experienced as punishing and frustrating objects instead of loving ones. Parts of these phantasy-constructed, frustrating parents are, again in phantasy, attacked in rage and then felt to return to haunt and persecute the child, confronting him and sometimes giving rise to nightmares and to terror.

To the young mind, such fragments are at times seen as returning 'in disguise', like a nightmare, suddenly confronting them during the day as they attempt to rationalize them into some small harmless object, which nevertheless strikes terror and anxiety into them. A particular horror is any small, fast-moving insect (particularly, for some, a spider or a snake). These may also act as a trigger to other equally primitive instincts of preservation and survivial more related to concepts of Jungian archetypal images of ancestral enemies — present since the dawn of mankind, but remaining the unconscious. In certain types, these ancestral and instinctual residues may release both panic and paralysis when a sudden movement of a certain object roots them to the spot or creates overwhelming panic. In certain countries, such small objects and insects are still a very real danger to the young child or baby, particularly the spider or snake. When the phobia takes the form of very small insects or animals, it is nearly always the unpredictability and sideways darting movements, after a period of immobility that inspires a sense of panic. Such feelings are often felt when suddenly confronted by a cockroach or crab.

The phobia may have been present for many years — often since adolescence or earlier. Perhaps at that time, because of an excessive phobia of becoming fat, there may have been an unhealthy preoccupation with slimming and weight loss. In others, the condition occurs in middle-life, from 35 onwards. Often, the phobic person has been apparently well, normal and able to take responsibilities until the onset of the illness. However, such people usually have a very rigid personality structure, with a stong sense of conscience and responsibility which has become overdeveloped over the years. In general they have been almost too normal, with a complete denial of any conflicts or problems in their own lives. Feelings of dissension or rebellion in any situation have never been openly admitted in the past, either at work or in the family. Ambivalence has been firmly suppressed over a long period, and only now, in later life, threatens to emerge, in spite of the strict controls. At the same time, the emergence is often indirect, so that becoming more human also leads to many bizarre fears and terrors as long-repressed feelings of love as well as resentment are finally brought into the open.

An unconscious battle is commonly present in phobic conditions — a fight between patterns of long-standing, rigid controls and personality make-up, conflicting with impulses to change, break out or break away and to develop. For once in their lives these individuals long to be tear-aways, to show that they too can be aggressive, rebellious and non-conforming — at least to some degree. But above all, what really matters is to show themselves that they can be a person in their own right — not caring quite so much what others think or may say about them. Such impulses occur quite naturally in the 40 year age group and also in later years, when there is a feeling that time is against them, and that soon it will be too late to emerge and that nothing is really more important than the personal expression of themselves.

This determination to emerge can also lead to anxiety, panic, and fear — a sense of pressure, of 'going mad', especially in a person who has previously always conformed. Sometimes it is more the family that expresses the fears once the individual member has decided on a course of action and is suddenly able to free himself from constrictions and earlier ties. But usually there is a conflict which is the cause of all the phobic's unconscious problems and pressures. Impulses to change and anger towards one of the parents felt to have been over-protective in earlier years are the causes of considerable resentment, ambivalence and childish rage. The awareness of such feelings may cause a mixture of both guilt and anxiety, and if the inner conflict is not resolved in a more healthy way than in the past it can easily lead to a state of acute and crippling agoraphobia.

In most cases of phobia the child-parent relationship has been excessively close, the child over-sensitive and identifying with the parents in order to please and placate, at the expense of his own individuality. A situation of fear is already present, and such attitudes of excessive identification are particularly common in a first or only child. Not infrequently, a phobia may develop to mimic a similar problem in one of the parents with whom there is an unhealthy, excessively close tie, in another attempt to ensure closeness and reassurance against loss of love which the child senses to be fragile.

More rarely, phobias are associated with a personality change which is not part of emergence, development and growth. There may be a history of head injury, epilepsy, or the condition may be due to a tumour. When phobia occurs due to an underlying organic illness, there is usually at the same time a deterioration generally, both mentally and physically, without the usual rigid personality patterns. In general, an organic cause of a phobic condition is very rare.

Agoraphobia

Agoraphobia is fear of open spaces. Usually it is an adult problem, more common in women than men. A similar fear occurs in the young adolescent with unstable schizophrenic tendencies, when there may also be fear of going out of doors for delusional reasons; here the condition is not typically phobic in origin.

The problem is a powerful sense of weakness and vulnerability, of exposure to danger, without protection and a feeling of being trapped whenever the individual is outside the security of the home. Acute anxiety is present particularly with a feeling of collapse, fainting or falling and ultimately of dying. Often there is a hysterical element present, a fear of making a fuss, or making a 'show', which hides strong exhibitionistic features of the problem. Usually the agoraphobic will venture outside the home with someone else to provide security and protection, but even then for only the briefest periods.

Outside, particularly wide open squares or roads, represents a threat; they must be crossed as quickly as possible, and always at their narrowest point. Any situation where the person is likely to be delayed or held up is a cause of renewed panic and fear — particularly any queue, traffic jam, or supermarket check-out point. Shopping, with having to wait at the till, is a cause of the typical mixed feelings of panic and aggression which can flair up in any queue or situation of frustration. Any delay means that they cannot make a quick getaway, leading to a sense of being trapped, with sweating, palpitations, and fear of either collapse, or aggressively attacking the person who may be holding up the queue. In short, part of the problem is a mixture of great impatience, the fear of violence, and loss of control. Generally, the underlying ego or personality is weak, with few reserves so that collapse seems always imminent.

Agoraphobia also occurs in small children when there is a fear of leaving home, particularly of leaving the mother alone — in case something happens to her. Such children also have the typical phobic feelings of insecurity and dependence, and often have a strongly ambivalent attitude towards the parent in question, with the usual aggression, that is not dealt with or acknowledged at the time, just pushed under the surface. In such cases the family has often contrived to make the phobic child both a victim or container of their own feelings, as well as the centre for their concern and family unity.

Deep within himself, the agoraphobic feels alone, depressed and exposed, with no protection, safety or security except when within the family home. He is totally dependent on another person — usually the spouse, sometimes a daughter or neighbour — and there is a return to infantile dependence.

The main feeling is one of abandonment and lacking any sense of security, as if it had never been present, although in the past these individuals have often been highly successful and confident. They cling to the home because of this sense of being so unprotected and vulnerable, as if near to collapse, unable to survive modern life, noise, and the demands of people, all of which both threaten and profoundly irritate them.

Recommended Remedies for Agoraphobia

1) *The Constitutional Remedy of the Individual*
Give this initially in the 200c potency whenever it can be clearly discerned.

2) *Aconitum*
This is best given for the acute case marked by fears of collapsing or dying if they go out. They are absolutely convinced about this so that fear, even terror, is a marked feature. Also use in those cases where acute fear has been the trigger to the agoraphobia. Use the high potency.

3) *Arnica*
Use when there is any history of acute shock or trauma which first provoked the phobic reaction. In such cases use in the 200c dilution. It is also indicated in those cases where there are marked feelings of weakness and fainting, and where the person is somewhat indifferent to others and just wants to be left alone — always provided that someone is not too far away. In such cases of near collapse or weakness use the 6c potency thrice daily.

4) *Arsenicum*
Indicated in those cases where is a combination of severe agitation, restlessness and phobia at the same time as a sense of paralyzing weakness, exhaustion and collapse. It is useful in acute cases which have such a symptom pattern. Use in the 200c potency.

5) *Aurum met.*
There is great intolerance of any traffic noise or the smell of petrol. Hypersensitivity to any external disturbances is marked, with a combination of irritability and depression.

6) *Natrum mur.*
The basic personality is always fearful, depressed and a 'loner'. There is often a chronic problem going back over many years with a dislike of people, noise and any disturbance of the daily routine, which varies little from day to day. Fresh country air is liked, but the worst possible situation is a busy, noisy seaside promenade. Always use the high potency 200c remedy.

7) *Platina*
The personality is always a difficult one to either like or relate to

because of the features of pride and superiority. But under the surface there soon emerge problems of depression and lack of confidence — especially in any situation of traffic, noise or people.

Claustrophobia

Claustrophobia is fear of enclosed places. As with all phobic conditions, security of the individual is weakly established, the ego feels vulnerable and unable to defend itself in the phobic situation. These individuals feel swallowed up, unable to escape, sometimes devoured and lost, never to reappear from what is experienced as an enclosing, strangling situation. Lifts, aeroplanes, middle-aisle seats, the undergound, or any form of travel with the exception of their own cars, are a threat and present a situation where they may become trapped. Often fear arises in any situation where they feel dependent upon another person — a neighbour stopping them for advice or a chat is similarly felt to block and control them, often creating anxiety. In any of these situations, physical symptoms are common, especially a feeling of collapse or fainting, sudden diarrhoea, giddiness or being unable to breathe.

Unconsciously, the claustrophobic feels trapped within himself by many of his own attitudes and his life-style. Often he feels trapped by his job, clothes, language and his role, as well as by the way others see him. The typical phobic conflict is invariably present — the wish to expand his personality and develop in certain areas conflicts strongly with impulses to stay put and remain stagnant in a safe womb-like existence, felt to be uncreative and restricting. They are not happy with their lives, and often feel that their illness and way of life has been more a form of death to their individuality than any form of real living. Faced with such a powerful conflict over many years, it is not surprising to see such terror created by the unconscious, distorting any vehicle of change or growth and learning into a danger. Buried alive within themselves, such personalities naturally fear being trapped and unable to get out of an external situation, which is really a mirror of their inner dilemma.

Such conflicts create a real terror of enclosed spaces, and constant attempts to avoid them. Always extremely dependent people, they also fear being trapped by dependent habits and addictions to food, alcohol and cigarettes — symbols of their need to lose and bury themselves in a relationship, habit or a job where their individuality cannot emerge. Such patterns of fear and dependency, present since earliest infancy, in one form or another have prevented them ever maintaining a truly giving and loving position — yet this is what they most value and seek, in spite of the fear which it also brings.

For the majority, all support, aggression, ability to cope and decision-making are left to the partner who is the strong one — able to work, travel and manage without fear. This division creates problems and tensions in the home, although these are usually well tolerated. For many, claustrophobia is not so much an illness as an aspect of the personality make-up, which can accompany the more severe agoraphobic state at times, so that a mixed phobic state exists. Apart from the immediate family, most people are avoided, particularly any superfluous contacts, in case they get 'caught up' in a debate or discussion. There is also great intolerance of heat, particularly any stuffy atmosphere, and the typical *Pulsatilla* need for open space and open air is common. They fear suffocation as much from an anaesthetic as from certain people or an over-heated room — hence the fear of tunnels, or anything that could collapse on them. Breathing is a vital preoccupation, and there are many similarities to asthma. Obsessional personality traits are common to both conditions; the asthmatic often feels trapped and shut in by wheezing and bronchial spasm.

The typical claustrophobic make-up is predominantly infantile. At home they are often charming, seductive, and witty and amusing. The problem is always with others who may arrive as 'intruders', and make demands, bringing about fear. Closeness is always avoided, and even in a good period there is a tendency to dart about like a frightened fawn, always shy, lacking in confidence and wanting to get away.

Recommended Remedies for Claustrophobia

1) *Argentum nit.*
The most important remedy — the person for whom this is indicated is weak, fearful of any enclosed situation and weak both physically and mentally. In any situation outside the home there is a fear of being trapped and unable to get free or away quickly enough. An end or aisle seat is always essential, and there is often a sense of tall buildings or narrow streets crushing or falling in upon them. Diarrhoea or the need to have the bowels open in a public situation is a constant and common fear. Heat in any form is oppressive in the extreme *Pulsatilla*. Use high potencies.

2) *Carbo veg.*
There is a combination of feelings of weakness and collapse generally and these are aggravated at the suggestion or thought of seeing others or going out. Panic feelings are marked. Use the 30c potency thrice weekly.

3) *Pulsatilla*

These personalities easily feel shut in and trapped, are in a panic and feel threatened by others whenever there is a situation where a demand may be made or they feel on show. Any public, closed in, hot and airless room or the underground or a lift is a threat, causing anxiety, as if they will faint or not be able to catch their breath or get away. At the same time, other people are needed, but only on their own terms and terrain. The typical, passive, tearful, changeable *Pulsatilla* personality must be present for the remedy to be effective. Despite their intolerance of heat or any clammy situation, they are rarely thirsty. Use the 200c potency.

4) *Sulphur*

There are deep-seated personality or mental disturbances present, so that any closed in situation involving others is a threat. These individuals need to control and create their own boundaries in any situation, and often have their own rules as to the interpretation of words and language. Withdrawal into a phantasy world is common and often accompanied by a poor memory, much confusion generally and feelings of unreality — hence the threat created by any 'enclosed' situation. Use the 200c potency. It may need to be repeated on several occasions during the treatment.

Fear of Eating Out in Public

Excessive anxiety is present in any situation where food and drink is taken in front of others — for example in a restaurant or open place. There is always an excessive awareness of others, and a sense of being both observed as well as a feeling of having to eat and being under pressure. Such eating is seen as a performance, and meets with strong unconscious resistance, so that the least mouthful or sip of food or drink is only swallowed with the greatest difficulty. There is a paranoid element present because of the powerful sense of being observed and watched by others, as if always under scrutiny and the centre of attention. Eating in such conditions nearly causes the hands to shake, and this tendency to shake is a common source of additional anxiety in case they make a mess or spill something, and create even more attention.

In spite of hunger, they often feel full after one mouthful, and are unable to take any more. It is as if the small child was being force-fed by an adult who insisted on them taking more from the cup, when the child himself wants to go more slowly and have a rest. Nothing must be left on the plate as this meets with disapproving glances or comments, yet the individual feels immediately full. This feeling of being full after one mouthful is a typical characteristic of *Lycopodium* and an indication to prescribe.

There is also the common feeling of being about to faint, especially if the room or restaurant is at all warm, and this often reinforces the anxiety of drawing attention to themselves — a feature of the strong need of approval. The great fear is of ridicule, collapse, choking, being looked at and judged in an eating situation, causing panic so that they have to leave. At the same time there is often a claustrophobic fear of being trapped and unable to leave the table. Such fears and preoccupations represent damage at the early mouth/oral development stage of the personality, so that everything is now dominated by the obsessional fear of eating, which causes a great deal of pain and anguish, and inevitably a further stunting of social development.

Recommended Remedies for the Fear of Eating Out in Public

1) *Lycopodium*
Always severely anxious in almost any situation, particularly a new one, which upsets the digestion — often days beforehand — worrying about it. These individuals always feel on show, that a demand is about to be made of them and that they are not prepared for it. They are intolerant of any change of mealtimes, of diet or delay whatsoever, provoking a sensation of emptiness and collapse. Use the 200c potency.

2) *Gelsemium*
The basic make-up is of over-sensitivity and wanting to be left alone, not being bothered by others or spoken to. Almost everyone irritates them and this leads to powerful critical feelings. These types dread being in public or looked at. The remedy has powerful eye representation or acts as a quite specific tonic action on the eye muscles, relieving fatigue and weakness. It has a value in strengthening weakness or paralysis of the eyelids — after a stroke, in the elderly, and in such diseases as myasthenia. But it also has strong emotional eye associations too and where *Gelsemium* is indicated, the personality also intensely dislikes being stared at, although at the same time they tend to be inquisitive and not to be adverse to look at others in what is often a critical and negative fashion. It is best used in the high, 200c potency, provided that the basic make-up is clearly present.

3) *Medorrhinum*
Any public situation of eating out poses a threat and is dreaded. The worst disaster is always anticipated and the evening seems interminable.

There are often overwhelming fears of dying if these individuals cannot escape the situation. The only situation where they feel more relaxed is at the seaside when such a meal may not only be tolerated but enjoyed. Use the 200c potency.

4) *Plumbum*
The make-up associated with this remedy is full of fears, especially of being attacked or poisoned by the food. Such types are very careful what they eat to the point of being obsessional, and they would never eat mushrooms in a restaurant. Severe constipation is a constant feature, with attacks of the most violent colic at times, and in general there is a lack of appetite and interest in food. Use the high 200c potency.

5) *Phosphoric acid*
The major feature here is the lack of energy and strength to go out, so that the thought of a meal out and meeting people causes dread.

6) *Silicea*
Timid, anxious, fearful of others, especially of being clumsy or awkward, these personalities feel weak, lacking in conversation and *savoir faire*. They feel paralyzed and the thought of a long drawn out meal is a nightmare. Use the 30c potency.

Fear of the Opposite Sex
This is not so much a phobia as a loss of confidence in the self which inevitably has its roots in infancy. The fear is one of rejection and hides a sense of failure and inadequacy, often feelings of hostility. There is sometimes a conviction that the parents preferred another sibling to them, so that they always feel somewhat unwanted or awkward whatever the situation. Such fears are common in adolescence until confidence and security are well established.

In adults, these fears often occur after the break-up of a marriage, when there may be feelings of depression or an adjustment to a new partner. Typical sexual problems which occur at such times are premature ejaculation or frigidity, and when present they cause additional anxieties in relationships or making new friendships. When such fears are present they cover up very strong feelings of interest and attraction for the opposite sex, and this may become a preoccupation to the exclusion of all else. Often the fears cover a sexuality that is too exciting to be tolerated or permitted, so that it is turned into a threat or felt to be overwhelming.

Ultimately, such fears are narcissistic in character; they are concerned with losing control or face, hurt in one's pride by feelings that have previously always been controlled and which are ultimately self-preserving rather than giving or sharing. Letting go in any situation becomes a threat because they may not be able to cope with it. When such problems involve the male, the woman is avoided because she becomes a threat to self-esteem, as are all other potentially creative, but enveloping situations, in either work or social areas.

Recommended Remedies for the Fear of the Opposite Sex
Such fear usually means that there is an exaggerated and often secret interest in the situation feared.

1) *Pulsatilla*
The *Pulsatilla* personality is always anxious and unsure of himself, lacking in confidence and maturity. At the same time they are anxious to please and to be liked. There is no lack of sexual interest or indifference; on the contrary, there is almost a preoccupation with sexual matters and possible relationships or liaisons. The main problem area is making the initial contacts — after that there is usually no great difficulty, and although the usual passivity and timidity is present, this does not pose any severe barrier. In any new situation, whenever these individuals feel themselves to be on display or if there is the possibility of a rejection, they panic. Use the 200c potency. (The remedy acts for approximately 2 months.)

2) *Ignatia*
The underlying problem is often that the personality make-up is a hysterical one, the fears sometimes provoked by the shock of grief or loss — perhaps the break-up of an earlier love-affair or engagement. There is a mixture of both interest and provocation together with severe panic and fear. Use the 200c potency when there is a history of loss causing the fears; if this is not clearly established use in the 30c potency thrice weekly.

3) *Calcarea*
There is a combination of weakness, withdrawal, shyness and rather sad indifference and passivity. Confidence is not the strong point of this personality, and he easily becomes irritable, even to the point of feeling ill when frustrated. The basic personality is often deeply disturbed — these types are obsessional, have difficulty knowing what to say, and are generally not very strongly orientated towards a physical relationship; sexuality is never very strongly developed. Always use the 200c potency.

10.

GRIEF AND LOSS

Mourning, grief and loss are an inevitable part of every human experience. Often they are deepening experiences in that every loss, even every disappointment is to some extent a development and prepares us for our own inevitable mortality and death at some time, teaching us the limitations of over-idealization. At the same time such grief emphasizes our vulnerability and the pain also reminds us that all life is change, that everything has a beginning and an end, that every gain, every new learning experience also entails a loss and is often at the cost of a much-cherished belief or position or conviction.

Life itself can be seen as a chain of grief reactions and ruptures with the past. It is also an opening of new doors and experiences, often of new relationships, but always they are inseparable from loss in some form or other. However life is viewed, optimistically or otherwise, from birth onwards there are inevitable disappointments beginning with the loss of the foetal state of bliss. Weaning, the break from the breast, relinquishing infancy for childhood is, in all cases, a form of loss and separation from the familiar, so that often such changes are accompanied by fear, anxiety and sadness. It is just such early infantile feelings that can also re-emerge in the adult state of grief and loss, with a repeat of grief for every state of loss and alienation that has ever occurred thoughout life from infancy onwards.

Some of the sadness felt at birthdays and the thought of growing older is also one of mild grief at no longer being a teenager. Similar feelings often occur on leaving school, getting married or reaching a particular age of, say, 30, 40 or 50. In all these situations there is regret for the past as well as a sense of relief and achievement. For many, fear of the new circumstances and the future is also present. But grief is part of everyone's experiences and every separation, even if temporary, from a person who is cared for is to 'die a little', so that, when looked at closely, grief and separation are inseparable from life and change itself.

Mourning and Grief

Mourning follows loss and is the normal grief reaction. Initially, there is a sense of shock and disbelief, often one of self-reproach and guilt: 'I should have been more thoughtful and understanding, I should have done more, been there, seen it all earlier, questioned the doctors more, given more, loved more and showed it more positively'. In fact what is being said is 'I should have been omnipotent and prevented death happening'! During this initial stage of shock and self-reproach, remedies as *Arnica* or *Aconitum* are invaluable when fear, collapse and shock are considerable; but always give *Arnica* initially. Feelings of rage and hostility can quickly follow the shock and disbelief, in particular towards the 'caring agents' — the doctors, nurses, the hospital or clinic to whom feelings of defeat and helplessness are directed. Such common hostility is also an expression of anxiety and reflects a projection of guilt onto others. But whatever the circumstances, even in a sudden fatal road accident, there is always some feeling of being personally responsible.

In some cases, the aggression released is not turned on the hospital, but more directly towards the lost person who is reproached. When this happens, the lost person is sometimes blamed for leaving without warning, for abandoning them at a most inconvenient and difficult time; or in other cases, for going first and leaving them behind. The sense of loss and abandonment is felt very acutely and is part of the feelings of being bereft. These feelings are indeed often experienced in infantile terms and language, to be followed by a third phase of disturbance, where depression is most marked.

The feelings of shock, reproach and guilt are often followed in this third period by a prolonged and overwhelming sadness, insomnia, depression, loneliness and a sense of emptiness and fear. Insomnia and weeping is very marked and during this time *Pulsatilla* is helpful, provided that the person can accept and is relieved by consolation. If not, and any form of consolation irritates and aggravates, give *Natrum mur.* There is an overwhelming sense that life is over and that it has no purpose any more. The grief-stricken person lives in the past, dominated by what they have lost and by fear and insecurity. There seems to be no hope of anything to look forward to except their own inevitable and imminent death. There seems no reason for living and, in severe cases, they only consider continuing to exist because of the children and because of the family, but not because of themselves and their own wishes. They often feel emotionally dead. It seems as if the source of all inspiration and hope is irretrievably lost and behind them.

Such feelings of despair, loss, loneliness, disorientation and sadness may last for many weeks and months, until suddenly there is a feeling of coming alive again and a realization that such despair is not what the lost person would have wished.

Failure to Mourn
Unless there is a total lack of caring for the lost person, an absence of the normal mourning reaction means that there is a denial and repression of the painful processes of grief and associated feelings because they cannot be admitted to. Whatever the reason, the person feels unconsciously that he must at all costs keep feelings of sadness and loss to himself. But this undeclared and denied grief cannot remain buried indefinitely, and must find an exit in one form or another since it is charged with considerable energy of feelings. Sooner or later the reaction surfaces often as a violent shock or delayed grief, or in other cases as an overwhelming 'anniversary' explosion of excess feelings.

In such cases of denial there may be a powerful physical reaction with the onset of a severe illness with sudden collapse. When there are hysterical tendencies the atypical illness that develops may sometimes resemble the final illness of the lost person. Frequently, such an illness may be incapacitating and limiting over a period of many months or years and remain totally mysterious until the cause is finally revealed, often by the family. One patient who came to me for treatment was very attached to a much-loved younger brother who had died several years previously; since that time the patient had never really been right, although there had been no overt reaction of emotion at the time of the death. In some cases, the denial of grief has been very serious and has resulted in the patient undergoing a whole gamut of investigations and tests; for some several explorative operations have occurred all without relief of symptoms or clarification of the roots of their malaise. In such cases there seems to be an element of masochism present as part of their guilt, and often aggression in the form of resentment at being exposed to so much potential pain.

In some cases the denial and the bizarre, often displaced symptoms which express underlying feelings, may become chronic and incurable. In others, the physical symptoms, unclear and long-standing, lead into a condition of depressive illness with an eventual total nervous break-down. The cost of the denial of mourning is therefore often considerable and the loss of health and vitality is great because of the amount of energy used to keep all feelings of loss beneath the surface.

In other cases mourning involves the loss of a still-born child or may follow a miscarriage or provoked abortion, with strong feelings of sadness and loss, often emerging many years later and especially when there are no other children.

Some Case Notes of Grief and Mourning

A woman of 35 came because her hair lacked bounce and vitality and was thinning markedly. The condition came on following the death of a much-loved brother killed on a motorway accident when on his way to see her. The evening of the fatal accident they were all very busy preparing for a holiday. He had telephoned asking whether he should come over on his motor-cycle. She had encouraged him to come and see them rather than go to the cinema with a girl friend. She — the patient — felt that she had persuaded him to come over and that the accident was partly her doing. As she talked of the accident she became increasingly tearful and depressed with an emergence of her feelings of guilt and self-reproach. There was a rapid improvement in her hair condition following treatment with *Ignatia*, but the underlying depression took several months to resolve. *Natrum mur.* gave the final relief, but not until many weeks after the presenting symptoms of hair problem had been completely resolved.

A woman of 55 lost her husband very suddenly. There was no normal grief, but from the start there was a refusal to eat and inability to sleep, with increasing agitation. The patient became increasingly disturbed and ill and was admitted to hospital. A month following the husband's death the wife had died in hospital, all attempts by medical and psychological means having failed.

A patient in her sixties came with problems of insomnia, exhaustion and weakness. It eventually emerged that she was with her husband when he had a 'coronary' at the wheel of their car on the motorway. The patient had come for help at a time of the anniversary of the accident two years previously. She became less depressed as she improved physically and one year later, having seen her monthly, she was fully recovered.

The husband of a patient in his early sixties with a history of manic-depression developed angina cycling uphill and this led on to a fatal heart attack. The wife became very depressed; she had never taken his complaints very seriously, had always correctly seen him as hypochondriacal and a man who would take to his bed at the least pain or symptom. She had always been the dominant one and pushed him hard in order to encourage him into activity. Following his death she felt very nervous and full of guilt. For many weeks she could not sleep in the dark or without someone else in the house because of nightmares. Many of these fears were infantile in origin, and following the husband's death she re-experienced many of the early anxieties of childhood and a revival of insecurities from this period. There was a good response to *Ignatia* and after one treatment the patient had regained her confidence.

Recommended Remedies for Grief and Loss

1) *Aurum met.*
This remedy is indicated for the very severe cases of grief where depression is such as to create a definite suicidal risk. The state of mind is very worrying for the family and often the individual cannot be roused, either from his depression or his determination on suicide. These patients are full of hopelessness and self-reproach, and cannot be consoled or reassured. Their determination is to end it all and they just want to be left alone to think quietly. There is often considerable agitation so that they walk up and down, planning how to commit suicide. At the same time they are easily irritable, unforgiving and full of resentments and indignation — feeling hard-done-by by life and fate alike.

2) *Arnica*
This remedy is indicated for the acute shock of grief and loss. There is a sense of weakness and exhaustion, of being 'all gone', sad, wanting to be alone and at peace. In general, where *Arnica* is indicated in the acute phase, the person concerned wants to be left alone and not spoken to. They are usually sad, fearful, anxious, and full of hypochondriacal, bruised feelings. There is a tendency to withdraw into silence, preoccupied and resenting questions or any form of contact or company.

3) *Baptisia*
This remedy is indicated when the patient is just exhausted, seems indifferent and only wants to sleep. There is total inability to think or to concentrate because of fatigue, confusion of thoughts and lack of energy. When opposed they are easily agitated, and only too soon afterwards sink back into an exhausted sleep.

4) *Ignatia*
This is the great remedy for grief. Usually it is best prescribed for dark-haired individuals. They are full of the typical *Ignatia* problems and contradictions. Changeable and over-sensitive to the extreme, these types are easily fearful and the remedy is especially valuable when the patient is unable to come to terms with the loss. Depression is marked,

but only since the loss. There is a tendency to be silent, withdrawn and morose. Often the sadness is carefully hidden and denied, yet there are also many sighs, regrets and tears. In general, there is a reluctance to share or discuss the pain, and because of this emotional lability and lack of control these patients are easily moved to laughter before sinking back into sadness.

5) *Naja*

This is another remedy for acute sadness to the point of suicide. These patients are exhausted, want to die, and torment themselves by their inability to bring back the lost person. Palpitations are very common. In general, they want to die from a broken heart and find the suffering all too much to take. When held or checked in any way they are quickly excited.

6) *Natrum mur.*

This is one of the major remedies for this condition. These patients are tearful and very depressed, often indifferent and usually worsened by any approach, especially of consolation. The main feeling is one of irritable hopelessness, aggravated by heat, the seaside and usually worse for cold wind or daughts which cause the eyes to water.

7) *Natrum sulph.*

This is recommended for depression where there is complete lack of concentration. These patients refuse to be spoken to or to share or discuss their grief. They much prefer to be left alone in solitude, and music always intensifies the grief. In general, the depression is worse on waking and improves towards evening.

8) *Phosphoric acid*

There is a combination of the most profound nervous exhaustion, apathy, prostration and debility. In general, these individuals are depressed after a shock and cannot think, concentrate or get themselves together in any way. Usually their prostration is worse from any form of effort whatsoever; they are often worse in the evening as the fatigue of the day catches up on them and they can only retire early to try and sleep, although this is usually fitful and troubled, giving no real rest.

9) *Sepia*

This is one of the most profound remedies and deepest acting. The key features are a grief marked by extreme fatigue, worse in the evening and as the day draws on. Irritability is also marked and accompanies a flat indifference to all, but is most noticeable towards those closest and most loved. Added to this is constipation and often a 'dragging down' backache or vague lower abdominal pains which serve to aggravate the sadness. Any contact with them usually meets with a rejection and leads to feelings of defeat and failure.

10) *Kali. carb.*

In contrast to *Sepia, Kalium carb.* is indicated when the patient cannot bear to be left alone and is usually highly nervous, full of fears and insecurity. Typically, there is insomnia, waking between three and five with anxiety, dread of the dark, and usually not falling asleep again until about six. Weakness is also present, but is less severe than the *Sepia* condition; these patients also lack the characteristic irritability associated with *Sepia*.

11) *Arsenicum*

This recommended for acute, agitated and restless states of mourning. These patients will not be reassured or calmed, needing others, but staying chilly and fearful and often very agitated.

12) *Lycopodium*

This is useful for hypochondriacal depressive states, worse in the afternoons about four. Insecurity and some form of gastric upset are very common.

11.

HYSTERIA AND STATES OF UNREALITY

There is a form of excessive emotionalism, with a marked display of feelings, which is often considerable and rarely passes unnoticed. In addition, there is often an overwhelming rush of feelings which swamp all others like a tidal wave. Such feelings sweep over the person completely so that, for instance, when the mood is one of laughter it takes over the whole of the person and everything shakes with excessive mirth and gaiety. When the mood is one of depression, every aspect of the person is sombre and every movement, gesture, grimace or remark is one of melancholy and sadness. There is usually a marked emotional lability with loss of control and frequent mood changes — either to tears or rage — but these are always overpowering and seem to dominate the whole personality, though often only fleetingly.

Jealousy is marked because there is always competition with others to a marked degree, stimulated by the very low level of self-esteem and the inflated view and extreme idealization of others. When these feelings of jealousy are not present there is commonly a sense of superiority and the 'rival' is devalued in their eyes, contrasting with the other idealized viewpoint. Both are equally disturbing attitudes and are distortions of the true personality of the other person. When there is marked jealousy, *Lachesis* may be the remedy that is most helpful.

Outbursts of violence and loss of control are not unknown and at times they may become frequent when the feelings of desperation become intense. The hysteric will stop at nothing to gain attention, feeling at the time that he has nothing to lose. At all costs, they must convince the other person of their needs and their hopelessness. Without the aid, admiration and understanding of the other key person with whom they are involved at the time, and who is felt to be much needed, there is a sense of panic, and the hysteric often feels that without this support and admiration, he will die, either physically or psychologically. The violence is justified because of the need to control the other person and to impress upon him the urgency of their desperate needs. Little attention and consideration, however, is paid to the needs and feelings of the other person, and this failure to be aware of the needs of others is a key narcissistic feature of the hysterical make-up; it is also a common reason for their being rejected by others, although the rejection is never as severe as the individual experiences it or fears it to be.

The emotional outbursts can quite suddenly swing from one mood to another and there is a change from relaxation and apparent happiness to a mood of absolute despair, loneliness, and a near suicidal state of defeatism. One moment, they can be shaking and white with rage, and few minutes later reappear blooming, happy, laughing, full of zest, and a picture of health.

These sudden mood changes reflect an essential part of their basic psychological instability. It is an aspect of their urgent need to impress upon and convince the other person of the intensity of their feelings. Because they have no confidence and no point of stability, the least expression of ambivalence or doubt by the needed person is taken as a rejection and a signal for the most desperate expressions of 'raw' emotions in an attempt to control and to avoid the dreaded rejection, abandonment and the loss of love.

Manipulation or emotional pressure and often emotional blackmail are common features. In order to avoid being left abandoned and unloved, manipulation is always a common feature. To prevent being abandoned, the hysteric has a natural flair for spotting areas of emotional weakness and vulnerability in others, and plays on these areas in order to avoid being left, as well as to constantly impress upon the other the harm that this would do were it to occur. The degree of manipulation varies with each person from acts of desperation and threats of suicide to just looking down, depressed and disappointed; at other times they may look attractive, irresistable and seductive, usually in a sexual way — the aim is always to manipulate the feelings of the other and to avoid being abandoned. Each mood and attitude varies from one moment to the next and is dependent upon the feedback and degree of emotional control and response from the other person.

This strategy to get their way can take the form of thinly veiled threats, tears, break-down or suicide. Feelings of failure, collapse, going to bed, or worse is always round the corner when the hysteric is thwarted or feels misunderstood. There can also be a sudden return to infantile ways — with wild demands, accusations and a complete loss of control and security — which is typically short-lived and dramatic. It is the primitive and early levels of phantasy concerning their own child parent relationship and parental sexuality which make for the childlike qualities of the hysteric. At the same time, the childish displays of pique protect them from the stresses of living in the present, because really they are only partly involved with life in the present as so much of them is bound up with and living in the past. In many cases they are most at ease with children since they relate so easily with them.

At the same time as living on their emotions and those of others, which they so often stimulate, these personalities often seem to confuse various types of emotions. This is because they rush headlong into emotional situations, being either over-idealistic or too intense. There is a constant tendency to get too involved with any emotional situation or relationship too quickly and prematurely, because they always feel that unless they create a good impression from the start they will lose face and admiration from others. They fear that this is their fate and often the most desperate attention-seeking devices are used to avoid being thought boring or trivial. Equally, there is a dangerous tendency to jump to conclusions, to think that they are being criticized, rejected and unloved. Loving and being loved is all-important to them, but their capacity to respond and to return love is often lacking.

Seduction and sexuality are common features of the hysterical personality together with flirtation and display. This seduction is present in language, body movement and expression. They can often relate most easily in a sexual way since it is at a non-verbal level and this avoids the vulnerability they feel when there is any form of intellectual or sensitive conversation. Except when in a manic mood, they often feel most at ease in a direct sexual situation.

The hysteric has a natural aptitude to use his body to its best advantage, and has usually done so since childhood. For example, in the case of the female hysteric, little girls use their bodies in movement and dancing to gain the attention of the father and often unconsciously to 'seduce' him away from the mother. It is in their sexuality and in body expression that they are at their most confident. Frigidity may be a problem, however, although this is not usually admitted to, and it is not at all uncommon for counterfeit orgasms to be created in order to placate and control the male if this is thought necessary. They are life's natural and highly skilled actors and actresses and this is apparent from the earliest age. Although the hysteric has no confidence in their own intellect and quality of their minds at any depth, they may show a great deal of skill in their choice of words, particularly those which evoke an emotional response, but usually the trend of thought has little real depth or breadth to it and is only part of their acting skill and manipulative potential.

The hysteric basically has no confidence in himself because he is unable to integrate or build up his inner resources from his experiences and inner relationships. Primarily, this is because they rarely listen or take in what others are saying, being intent on giving a good impression, avoiding a rejection and controlling and manipulating others. Experiences in any depth tend to be rare because of their deep mistrust of themselves. Since most of the time they are acting a part or a role, as they think others would like them to be, this contrived expression of themselves makes for a minimal development of knowledge, experience and wisdom. There is a tendency not to stay put in any situation to form a stable relationship and for much of the time their minds are elsewhere, jumping on ahead to something new, or calculating how to avoid an imagined rejection in the present.

Only when they are in a manic mood is there any confidence at all in themselves, and because it is manic, it is inevitably short-lived, based on an over-inflation of the ego and is usually a flight from depression. Such apparent confidence is all too often just another part of the appeal and part of the seduction that leads to true confidence in themselves as individuals.

Because they have no confidence in themselves, they are worried by ageing, their appearance and their weight. In fact they usually spend enormous periods of time on their looks to ensure a good presentation, and they often look very youthful. But this does little to lessen their fear of ageing, as they feel that looks and apparent youth are their only major asset. They themselves have little time for the elderly, feeling that they have little to offer them, and this may account in part, for their fear, of ageing.

Hysterical personalities have little time for the elderly unless they are part of the child-parent triangle, when there is often a peevish, clinging-dependent/rejecting relationship. They hate the thought of any physical decline, will go to any lengths to look young and to avoid ageing, although in their own eyes they are always looking for telltale signs, fearing it and seeing it in themselves and others. Because the main force of their energy is directed at people of their own age group or younger, with whom they have the most intensely ambivalent relationship, the elderly are either avoided or shunned as being useless and irrelevant; yet they pose a threat to them as well because it reminds them of their inevitable mortality.

Their ability to think either in depth or creatively with any originality tends to be extremely low. Much of this is because of their infantile attachement to what others think of them, and to dramatization, both of which go against new and original ideas because everything has to be planned, thought-out, contrived and predictable.

At the same time, there is nearly always an *excessive* infantile attachment to one of the parents, either by actually living near them or with them, or by being obsessed with talking about and preoccupied with them. The excessive infantile attachment is part of the unconscious, hysterical personality dynamic, the need for a parental figure to love them and yet through whom they can control, relive and express earliest babyhood and childhood needs again. The actual childhood was often frustrated and damaging for many complex family reasons, but basically most of the hysteric's problems are internal or imagined and, in most cases, there has been no acute, clear-cut, physical or psychological trauma to account for their problems. The parents may not actually even be alive, but the tie is there just the same, and comes out constantly in conversation. The link is nearly always strongly ambivalent, in terms of right- and wrong-doings, yet despite the criticism, they are quite unable either to forget the hurts, or to detach themselves from the parent. This strong continuation of the parent-child relationship, often encouraged by the parents, usually leads to an early loss of friendships. Sometimes the hysterical attachment is resented or is carried over to some other area of life, such as at work where a father-figure or a mother-figure is found to complain about, or to adapt, and to again limit experience and to recreate an unresolved infantile pattern of attitudes and relationships. Usually such outside relationships are short-lasting, and after a few weeks or months someone new is found to play the role.

These are life's eternal children, as if living in an eternal pantomime in which they are playing 'Peter Pan', never growing up fully, never reaching maturity and never really feeling that they are able to give. Their lives are sadly marked by weakness, always fearful, always insecure, lacking in confidence and fearing the least decision or responsibility in case it should lead to further isolation and alienation.

Recommended Remedies for Hysteria

1) *Argentum nit.*
This is recommended for hysterical types dominated by fear, unable to relax and spending their lives in a hurry, for no obvious reason other than a sense of time passing too quickly and being under pressure. Heat in any form is intolerable to them and worsens the frequent tendency to nervous diarrhoea. There are many obsessional phobic features, especially a feeling of being 'drawn' by water or towards the edge of heights.

2) *Asafoetida*

This is useful in mild hysterical conditions with a marked tendency to fainting at the least emotion. They are always very nervous however, and this contributes to their frequent digestive upsets, especially flatulence.

3) *Belladonna*

A combination of fear and anxiety worsens the typical problems of excitement which are marked by obvious redness and heat. In a hysterical crisis there may be some violent behaviour with a tendency to strike out. There are always much worse for restraint, for being held or touched, in fact, for any sudden movement, massage or jarring motion. In addition they are sensitive to the least draught of cool air and an open door can lead to a sudden torrent of complaints.

4) *Calcarea*

There is weakness of muscles as well as of concentration. Slow in everything, they often take a long time to grasp the point so that there is often confusion worsened by their lack of concentration and being generally preoccupied. They are usually chilly, even on the warmest day, and easily become hypochondriacal. Because they are so taken up with trivial detail and the obsessional preoccupation with irrelevant matters, they are never clear about whatever is under discussion. Chilly, yet sweating, especially about the forehead, the mind participates in the general lack of tone and flabbiness.

5) *Coffea*

Excitement and agitation is present to an extreme degree, with marked over-sensitivity as well as great changeableness of mood and feelings. The extremes of mood are similar to the symptoms associated with *Pulsatilla*, but the symptoms differ in the general improvement by heat or warmth which is in direct contrast to those of *Pulsatilla*. There is a common tendency to toothache which, paradoxically, is better for cold air.

6) *Gelsemium*

Sleepy slowness, exhaustion and laziness are the hallmarks here, with a wish to be quiet, left alone and at peace — not disturbed in any manner. At the same time they are full of fears, lacking confidence, especially before an examination. At other times they can be in a state of over-excitability, out of control, especially after any emotional shock or pressure. On such occasions they seem to collapse, unable to cope with everyday pressures other than by a reaction of hysterical protest and fear. After a crisis there may be a period of 'nervous hoarseness' or sometimes complete loss of voice with laryngeal paralysis, the legs also weak and trembling.

7) *Hyoscyamus*

There is a deep disturbance with depression, inability to think or concentrate, full of fears and phobias. Periods of hysterical over-activity alternate with prostration, collapse and exhaustion. The symptoms are always worse at night on lying down as they are during the menstrual flow.

8) *Ignatia*

This remedy is indicated when the individual is full of contradictions and quite contrary in all respects. He is irritable, changeable and worse for grief, but the whole emotional spectrum is unstable. In particular, they are full of paradoxes — a pain in the side is better for coughing rather than worse as might be expected; the sore throat is better for swallowing water and is not aggravated by it; in general, rigors, chills or shivers are better for being uncovered rather than for being warm; also their common problem of piles is improved by walking rather than through rest as is usual.

9) *Kali. carb.*

Depressed and fearful, especially of the dark or of being left alone, these individuals lack confidence in many areas. Weakness is a problem both mentally and physically, and the upper eyelids are often characteristically swollen. There is great exhaustion, partly because of all their conflicts, worries and fears. There are many contradictions and uncertainties in this personality, and like *Calcarea* they are rather overweight, round in build but without the excessive sweating. Often they feel worse for chill and damp but are also intolerant of heat, especially central heating or a dry office atmosphere. Typical physical features are the very common problems of chronic catarrh and sinus infections.

10) *Moschus*

This remedy is indicated for the manipulative and over-dramatic of hysterical pattern. There are violent outbursts of anger, tears, uncontrollable giggles, or at other times attacks of palpitations or sudden fears. A ball or sensation of a lump in the throat is frequent as are hysterical cramps in the abdomen or severe headaches. A characteristic feature is that of one cheek burning hot, the other being cold and pale. There is also much preoccupation with sexual matters to the exclusion of all else, usually at a purely phantasy, non-involvement level. Like all else about the symptoms associated with this remedy, relationships tend to be brief, intense and dramatic. In this respect they are of value in certain adolescent hysterical behaviour and emotional hysterical problems.

11) *Platina*
Arrogance, pride and conceit are the main features of this haughty type of hysterical make-up, which is all too often a simple defence against profound feelings of inadequacy, failure and lack of confidence. Often depressed, they are also irritable and fearful and this is increased by the frequent tendency to piles or a sensation of a tight band around the head or body. At times, there is also an odd, disturbing sensation that their body is enlarged in some area — the hand or arm often — and that others are as if dwarfs beside them.

12) *Pulsatilla*
Pulsatilla is associated with intense compliant sympathy and the need for attention in the individual. Everything is marked by change, from tears to laughter to anger and spiteful rage. Reassurance is constantly required and consolation always brings a sense of calm and understanding for a brief time, until there is another crisis. Heat in any form cannot be tolerated and always worsens the fears, the indigestion and the weakness. The menstrual periods are always a problem, irregular and unpredictable, never really well established since adolescence, and at such times the sexual preoccupations and anxieties are increased.

13) *Valerian*
This is one of the best remedies for a severe hysterical state with many physical symptoms and confusional ideas, often worst for rest yet aggravated by exertion. There may be a paralytic hysterical state involving a limb or any part of the body. A feeling of being dissociated or floating is common and gives the impression of levitation. The mind is full of confused ideas to the extent that at times these individuals are unsure of their own identity.

12.

INSECURITY, SHYNESS AND IMMATURITY

Personal confidence and security is basic to every aspect of being and living. Without it, every moment, every meeting, every new aspect and moment of life becomes a threat rather than a challenge and a joy. Confidence is usually present from earliest childhood and gives that sense of independence, strength and certainty that is so common in every healthy child. This psychological stamina takes origin and foundation in a stable family life and a close relationship within the home, giving self-reliance and a certainty which is the basis of all security throughout life. Only when it is built on wish-fulfilment or phantasy is security weak and fragile, without substance.

Confidence and security between the couple is not necessarily built up on a marriage certificate, as more and more young people realize, but only from a basically similar relationship of mutual sharing and trust. Security comes not from a job, savings, material achievement or success, but only from a deep sense of continuation within the self, giving a sense of survival and strength whatever the pressures and threats.

Insecurity
This is best defined as a sense of weakness and vulnerability — a feeling of being defenceless in a social situation which involves contact, meeting or talking with others. This varies from the situation of a sudden visitor — a neighbour calling, a member of the family staying over Christmas — to an invitation to a local reception or theatre party. Any time when there is the possibility of having to express an opinion, make a contribution or share an interest is turned into a potentially traumatic situation. When the individual is able to forget himself through contact with someone younger, who seems less of a threat, has problems of insecurity himself, or is able to put him at ease or stimulate his interest — he can then forget himself for a while, but usually only

for a temporary period, as fear and insecurity are never far away.

The inability to forget the self-image is a key cause of all insecurity and much of the time the self is under a siege of self-criticism by a tormenting conscience. Whatever is done or achieved, said or thought is constantly under scrutiny and criticism — as if by hypercritical parents — really an aspect of the ego and self. Often the real parents may have been critical or rigid in earlier years — through rarely to the extent of the tyrannical conscience — and in later years they have usually mellowed considerably, so that there is little resemblance between the actual parents and the critical aspect of the personality. The excessive self-awareness creates much of the tension and because of a tendency to criticize and to compare with others, problems are always highlighted whenever a social relationship is present.

Such a personality feels unable to defend himself against any real or supposed slights or criticisms, feeling at the mercy of others. Often all strength is felt to be lacking, though resentment is strong and can rarely be exteriorized. Meeting others, particularly anyone new, creates jelly-like shaking and quiverings from fear and the anticipatory need to prove themselves and to be acceptable to the new person. This need to prove themselves acceptable, yet the fear of being in the forefront, always causes anxiety and anguish. In general, emphasis is placed on strength, success and achievement, often power, intelligence and looks — all the things they feel they lack and envy — but rarely on sensitivity, caring or the ability to listen.

Aggression is feared not only in others, but most of all in the self where it cannot be allowed at any cost since the individual does not trust himself in any situation, including an aggressive one, fearing lack of control over such powerful feelings. This constant denial of aggression leads to insecurity and weakness, since they fear to show any anger or dissension whatsoever, so that arguments are rare. The lack of control and fear of both anger and disapproval does not prevent them from behaving in a tyrannical way to anyone in a dependent position, when no threat is posed. Such behaviour is often present in private, and contributes considerably to the insecurity.

There is a common tendency to make comparisons, and competition is a marked feature — often dominating all other aspects of their relationships. Such feelings are particularly strong, because at the same time as making such comparisons, they also devalue themselves. There is a tendency to idealize others, and the qualities which are lacking in themselves or not admitted to or allowed expression are both admired and envied in others. An artificial gulf is thereby created which adds considerably to insecurity and a feeling of difference and inadequacy.

Such feelings of inferiority, failure and uselessness undermine and invade the fabric of the personality. There is a feeling of being unable to reach or live up to such impossibly high standards — set largely by phantasy images of the parents, which the infant feels he can never meet and which get carried over and recreated again by projection into others. A typical 'Catch 22' situation is created — running away from contact with others, yet lonely and even more weak and inadequate without them. The intrinsic masochism, coupled with the overvaluation of others, creates and recreates the problem of shame and failure — whatever the successes and achievements in reality — and there are rarely any long-term feelings of strength or adequacy.

Such insecurity may be linked to a specific situation such as giving a speech or going for an interview, especially whenever there are feelings of being on display or judged. Success is all-important, a measure of being loved and accepted, and what impresses them most in others and logically most impresses others in their turn. Such success is needed almost as a thing outside the self; it allows the possibility of being able to impress others and to capture their esteem and admiration. When they do occur, such successes always give a welcome, though temporary respite from the old and familiar patterns of self-negation and criticism.

Recommended Remedies for Insecurity

1) *The Constitutional Remedy of the Individual*
This the most important initial step in treatment. It is recommended that it be given in high potency of at least 200c. This remedy must match the predominant psychological picture as well as the physical make-up and general physiology. Prescribing must be accurate to have an effect, and failure often increases any underlying lack of confidence and co-operation.

2) *Aconitum*
Use this remedy whenever there is a clear-cut precipitating cause of acute fright — as with a near drowning, a fall or accident, in some cases a family argument or break-up which has provoked terror and fear in a sensitive child. It is only indicated when there was no physical injury at the time. The acute fear which triggered the insecurity may have occurred many years in the past — the time scale is not important in the homoeopathic prescription.

3) *Arnica*
Arnica should be given in all cases where there is a history of injury,

often accompanying fright or possibly the fear or danger of death. The combination of physical injury and fear is the indication — for example, a severe fall in the playground at school with stitches and a period of treatment in hospital, or involvement in a car accident.

4) *Ignatia*

Use *Ignatia* only when problems have followed a definite and clear-cut history of grief — for instance, a child has never been the same since the mother died, completely lacking in self-confidence, yet failing to show any outward signs of grief or loss at the time.

5) *Natrum mur.*

This is one of the major remedies and best used in the high potency of 200c. The principle indications are general nervousness and excessive self-control with tension, the rigid avoidance of others and a general lack of naturalness and ease whatever the situation.

6) *Phosphorus*

This remedy is indicated for the personality that is outgoing, gregarious, popular and likes and needs others. At the same time there is always fear — often inexplicable — and powerful needs of reassurance.

Shyness

This is a most intense and painful form of insecurity, beginning in early adolescence; it can change meeting people or any unfamiliar situation into one of agony, almost persecutory in intensity and avoided whenever possible. Shyness is an acute, unpleasant form of self-awareness, discomfort and embarrassment, marked by a sense of being awkward, tongue-tied and incompetent.

Such feelings may be triggered by almost any other person — and even the thought of a meeting is sometimes sufficient to cause acute anxiety. Whatever the situation, there is a general sense of having one's back to the wall and of being constantly criticized and looking ridiculous, as is common to all problems of insecurity. Embarrassment is felt to be a cruel blow of fate, and the individual would do anything to avoid making a 'show', yet he feels unable to do so, constantly recreating awkwardness and shyness to this extreme degree, whatever the relationship or meeting.

Shyness is common to some degree in all teenagers during adolescent formative years. It is often more severe in girls, but present in both sexes. It makes itself known in the typical adolescent feelings of being a child without an adult body, invariably insecure — as much from lack of experience as for any other reason. A secure background can do much to build up the necessary confidence to avoid excessive shyness. By maximizing the richness of contacts and experiences and limiting the intrusion of parental problems and anxieties into growth experiences, many of the problems of shyness can be overcome, especially when independence is encouraged. A sense of shame and guilt is always closely linked to the typical adolescent preoccupation with sexuality and phantasy and, like anything else occurring at this time of development, it is extreme and excessive as well as being secret and hidden.

The similarity to a paranoid illness and magical thinking is apparent, but only rarely and in severe cases is there a break with reality leading to a frank schizophrenic problem. The secret sexuality is the main problem and responsible for much of the shyness and blushing; this also contains a secret signal of sexual attraction, present at an instinctive level and therefore not consciously controllable. To his dismay, the sensitive adolescent finds that whatever he does he is unable to avoid drawing attention to himself — either by keeping in the background or by his shyness, so that attention is constantly thrust upon him to a most unwelcome degree. This attention is always one of the most dreaded aspects of shyness. Inevitably, the unconscious needs for display and attention occur whatever the conscious mind dictates.

Much of the preoccupation with being looked at is nothing more than a hidden desire to look and the gratification of this overwhelming desire is paid for by feelings of shame and being looked at themselves. Such looking always contains a sexual element and motivation — hence the guilt and awkwardness. Because the voyeuristic needs are so strong and compulsive, so too shame is kept to the fore by a morbid sense of embarrassment. The very blushing seems to spell out sexual awareness and knowledge and to make public their thoughts and preoccupations in this area. The classical conflict of insecurity develops between exhibitionistic impulses and the need to draw attention and to be noticed, conflicting with the pain and sensitivity of the shame or shyness — for both are inseparable.

As already mentioned, there may be a thin line between insecurity, shyness and self-consciousness and the more severe schizoid disturbance of additional withdrawal and bizarre behaviour, a tendency to live increasingly in a make-believe world with all the symptoms of normal adolescent shyness and preoccupation increased, and at the same time denied and buried within the psyche. It is only when so much energy is turned inwards that the more severe schizoid disorders may occur, and their treatment is more difficult.

Recommended Remedies for Shyness

1) *The Constitutional Remedy of the Individual*
See the note in the chapter on anxiety.

2) *Pulsatilla*
Usually works best in a person of fair appearance, with a tendency to be non-aggressive and yielding in nature, with only occasional outbursts of anger and impatience, since these types agree far too easily. There is always intolerance of heat, which worsens the shyness and feelings of self-consciousness. A tendency to be very variable and changeable is the other key feature to accurate prescribing and good results. (*Pulsatilla* is one of the most effective and rapid remedies when accurately prescribed.)

3) *Nitric acid*
This remedy works best in those of dark complexion. There is a combination of shyness, anxiety and often depression. Many of the problems are often worse in the evening. There are usually problems occurring at a physical level in one of the orifices — for example mouth ulcers or blisters, pain in the anal region or haemorrhoids, or problems with the ears — perhaps a chronic eczema.

4) *Lachesis*
This is indicated for the more profoundly disturbed personality, with deep brooding problems of jealousy and mistrust, causing a shyness and yet accompanied by an aggressive component that is disconcerting. They are shy, unhappy people, ill at ease with others, even out of place. All symptoms tend to be worse in the morning and after sleep.

5) *Sulphur*
For the person that seems to be untidy, both physically and emotionally. The personality is often withdrawn and caught up in confused, often rather weird thinking, seems not to need others, so that their shyness is in a feeling of being caught out, of embarrassment and how to get away from others who make them feel awkward and are felt to be intruders in their phantasy world.

Immaturity
Immaturity of attitudes in some areas is common to everyone and reflects areas of the self where infantile needs and narcissism are still present in the adult personality. The immature personality has failed to

develop fully and still retains, in many areas, an infantile way of perceiving the world, reflecting in predominantly self-centred childish attitudes. This is apparent in the individual's perception and judgement of others and the way that life's experiences are received, understood and responded to. There is often a curious child-like quality to the person, both psychologically and often physically, so that they invariably look younger than their years — which is often over-important to them — as well being young in mannerisms and relationships. This explains the frequent bouts of jealousy or competition with a younger person, sometimes a daughter or child. Infatuations may occur, always with a young object of admiration, which soon degenerate into childish anger or outbursts.

The immature person is still the attention-seeking child — self-orientated, demanding with a stunting of normal development, so that a natural sense of masculinity or mature feminity fails to develop. Parents are frequently clung to in an infantile way and every aspect of the personality is involved and held up by this childish perception of the world. Others are seen as adults and as parental figures — able to cope in a complicated, incomprehensible adult world. The immature position is invariably one of feeling out of touch with everyday problems as the individual compulsively relives his childhood impressions of reality, and whatever the adult experiences, it seems to do little to promote reality or growth.

Recommended Remedies for Immaturity

1) *The Constitutional Remedy of the Individual*
See the note in the chapter on anxiety.

2) *Tuberculinum*
It is often necessary to give the nosode at least once in order to stimulate psychological maturity. In particular, it is helpful when there is general restlessness, weakness and anxiety. It is indicated especially when there is any history of chest weakness or any history at all in the family of either T.B. or chronic chest problems. It is best given in the 200c potency and should not be repeated for a year. The failure to mature is at least in part due to emotional restlessness which makes learning from experience minimal.

3) *Baryta carb.*
This is a similar remedy for retarded psychological maturity which is useful at an early stage in treatment, particularly when there is not the

history of individual or family chest weakness related to the *Tuberculinum* remedy, when it can often act as a first stimulus to growth.

4) *Silicea*
This one of the best remedies when there is a stunting and a weakness both psychologically as well as physically. There has been an arrestment of growth and maturity which leaves the person weak and vulnerable. Sweating is often profuse, especially of the feet, and is a measure of the constant loss of energy from the body.

5) *Arnica*
Use *Arnica* in high 200c potency at least once in the treatment, especially if there is any history of previous trauma — even a precipitate, traumatic or Caesarian birth is an indication for this as the blockage to maturity may have its roots since that time.

6) *Thyroid (Glandula thyroidea)*
Use this remedy in low potency if there is any indication of stunted physical and metabolic growth accompanying the immaturity.

7) *Calcarea*
The *Calcarea* make-up is nearly always immature because of the inherent weakness and tendency to withdraw. Weakness, exhaustion and water retention are marked. Almost everything in life seems too much effort, whatever its appeal.

13.

INSOMNIA

Insomnia is one of the commonest emotional and physical disturbances seen by every general practitioner. It is extremely common and at least a quarter of all patients seen by the doctor are quite routinely taking a sedative on a regular basis. The sedative-habit has often begun in hospital, after an operation or a confinement or any illness when the patient has stayed for a few days under treatment. Many patients are routinely sedated in hospital for the benefit, in most cases, of the nursing night staff, rather than for the needs of the individual patient, and often against their wishes. Following a period of hospitalization, it often takes the patient several weeks to return to a non-drugged sleep once confidence has been re-established, and some never achieve this independence again.

On other occasions, the habit has been caused by a period of stress and pressure, causing wakefulness, the doctor then giving routine sedation and reassuring the patient that these drugs do no harm and that they can be taken, with some discretion, quite safely on any future occasion of worry or mild insomnia.

In other cases, it is common for a supply of sedation, prescribed for one member of the family to be passed around and shared by others. The remedy is often well known by name, prescribed on repeat prescription, and considered 'safe'. It is also perfectly well know that this is exactly what would be prescribed for them at the busy surgery. So the habit spreads, as does the dependence, throughout the whole family.

In most cases, insomnia is due to anxiety and pressures with the consequent inability to relax in bed. There may have been a shock or illness within the family, a period of grief and loss, or perhaps nursing and caring for a sick and demanding relative has drained all reserves and left the individual exhausted and unable to relax or sleep because of it. Money and work problems are other frequent causes, as are crises within or at the ending of a relationship or marriage.

Such emotional problems cause an over-active mind and when sleep comes, it is often troubled, with disturbing dreams and bewildering, chaotic nightmares, so that the individual wakes exhausted and unrefreshed. Before an examination or speech or any important, new and unfamiliar occasion, anxiety and fear may predominate and undermine rest.

Physical problems such as asthma, arthritic pain, indigestion, angina, coughs, sinus problems, shortness of breath and pain in any form may also disturb sleep, creating anxiety and exhaustion in addition to the underlying physical distress.

For some, insomnia is a long-standing problem, much as constipation, and sedatives are taken, much as are the purgatives and laxatives for the bowels. There are generally several different varieties used, and these may often be repeated during the night and at the whim of the patient, rather than on the advice and prescription of the doctor. Such drugs give little real relief or satisfying depth of slumber, and in many cases they have become a habit with problems of drug dependency and a chronic state of tension, unease and weariness which nothing seems to ease or to relieve.

The over-active child is a special problem, whose behaviour is often provoked by a precipitate birth and marked by exhausting over-activity during the day, rarely resting or playing at anything for more than a brief period. The child is constantly here, there and everywhere in need of constant supervision. Sleepless at night, such over-activity is also exhausting to the parents who then likewise suffer from insomnia because of the constantly disturbed rest. Homoeopathy is often needed in such cases for both the disturbed child and also the worn-out parents.

Recommended Remedies for Insomnia

1) *Lycopodium*

This is recommended for insomnia due to an over-active mind where thoughts and ideas about the future whirl around causing anxiety and tension, most of them anticipatory in character. These patients are often tired at about 8.00 p.m. and then cannot sleep when it is time to. They often fall asleep in the early hours and wake exhausted after an unrefreshing sleep.

2) *Chamomilla*

There is an overwhelming tiredness and somnolence during the whole of the day, including meal times. Generally, they are restless and there seems to be no established sleep pattern. Useful for severe jet lag insomnia.

3) *Gelsemium*
There is an inability to get off to sleep because of general restlessness and over-activity of the mind. The sleep is always light.

4) *Ignatia*
The sleep is disturbed and restless, marked by sighing and nightmares.

5) *Cocculus*
This is indicated for the insomnia of exhaustion and over-tiredness as may follow nursing a sick relative. The individual is worn out by lack of sleep and, when it is possible, he finds he cannot wind down sufficiently to get off to sleep.

6) *China*
Usually there is a state of sleepy exhaustion most of the day with agitation and the inability to fall asleep at night. This remedy is also useful when the insomnia follows a period of excessive work and worry.

7) *Arsenicum*
This is indicated for insomnia that begins in the early hours after midnight. Having fallen asleep, the insomniac wakes up suddenly, often with anxiety at 1.00 a.m.

8) *Kali. carb.*
There is a state of chronic exhaustion and fatigue, with waking between 3 and 5.00 a.m. and the inability to fall asleep again, or at least until just before they are due to wake. In the morning they feel absolutely worn out.

9) *Pulsatilla*
This is useful when the person sleeps with his arms above his head. In bed he is restless, waking in the morning hours, tossing and turning, too hot in bed and cold when uncovered. There is a tendency to have a warm drink of milk, a biscuit or some other light snack and then to fall asleep.

10) *Silicea*
This is useful for restless insomnia with sleep-walking, talking in the sleep, nightmares, hot flushes and palpitations. Anxiety and drenching

night sweats add to the discomfort and agitation.

11) *Coffea*
This is useful for insomnia due to excessive tea or coffee drinking. The person is wide awake until 3.00 a.m., thinking, the mind full of ideas and worries. There is then a light, troubled and restless sleep, often with a disturbing dream or nightmare.

12) *Thuja*
The patient is exhausted but cannot sleep. He feels hot and dry, and when sleep finally comes he is awakened by dreams of falling or of heights. He wakes up completely exhausted and unable to face the day.

13) *Lachesis*
There is drowsiness all day, especially after meals, yet they remain wide awake at night. On waking up, they are always worse and any problem is paradoxically worsened by sleep.

14) *Lac deflor*
There is a restless insomnia, with drowsiness throughout the day and catnaps; also an intolerance of milk or allergy to it.

15) *Opium*
This is recommended in cases of restless insomnia; the individual is over-sensitive to the least noise and absolutely exhausted and sleepy during the daytime, falling asleep at the least opportunity.

16) *Plumbum*
This is useful for insomnia from an over-active mind which is full of imaginative ideas and phantasy. Spasms of colicky pain are frequent.

14.

MOOD SWINGS AND MANIC-DEPRESSIVE ILLNESS

Abrupt changes of mood occur readily and naturally from earliest infancy onwards; they can be easily observed in the very youngest child as the frustrations of living, having to wait etc., create pressures and disappointments, anger and pain.

For many the combination of particularly difficult social problems and, say, freak weather conditions will create chaos where the most saintly temperament is hard put not to swing into frustration and rage at some point. Packed trains, buses and roads; getting to work and then home; often tiring nights away from the family in hotels with disturbed sleep, these are the factors which add to the general weariness and fatigue. During the day, reorganization, anxiety about job security and the future generally, creates further tension for many and is increasingly becoming a familiar facet of working life under the economic crisis. All too often the individual is used as a pawn in a political power game or show of muscle and the uncertainties as to outcome and resolution of such manoeuvres adds to the general fatigue and irritability.

For the woman, such problems are heightened at the time of the menstrual cycle when all emotions and feelings are more volatile and closer to the surface. In such a situation, the 'stable norm', without a swing into exasperation or anger may be less healthy than the uncontrolled curse and outburst. The person who bottles up his tension may be the loser in terms of physical and emotional health.

Such reactions to provocation, largely dependent upon external pressures and frustrations, are in direct contrast to those where mood swings are a way of life. For these individuals, such variations have been present as long as can be remembered and troughs of underlying depression seem to be inevitable. In addition, such mood swings always differ in one very important aspect from those of the outraged commuter or executive about to be 'phased out'. There is almost invariably a total lack of humour, banter or sense of the comic concerning their situation. Deadly serious and intense, they see problems and difficulties as grim, seeming to almost feel them more personally than others. For many, whatever the problems, however inconvenient the weather or the strikes, however intense the anger and outrage, some element of humour is never really far away and this helps to avoid any loss of perspective. Indeed, there is often a sense of 'occasion', of sharing brought about by an awkward situation.

For the less stable personality, there is none of this; everything is seen as deadly grim and the idea of a joke being cracked at the height of a crisis seems to them to be nothing but incomprehensible madness. Primarily this is because of their severe self-centredness and associated panic feelings at any change of routine. Much of the time, the 'mood swinger' feels that he is only just holding on as it is, and to have to bear these extra burdens and to laugh or joke about them is beyond him. Vulnerable, cursing internally, except during the high phase when his outpourings are almost inappropriate or excessive, he is without grace or humour, quite unable to find any relief in a sense of ridicule or 'all-in-it-together' feeling. Sadly, this attitude is upheld throughout life.

When there is no immediate crisis, mood changes occur nevertheless. Perhaps more subtle, but still recognizable, these types change from buoyancy and optimism at the least piece of positive news, to a mild 'downer' when it is not so good or slightly disappointing. All of these swings can vary daily in degree and frequency, and a delayed period, a birthday, the weather, or an anniversary, in fact almost anything can be turned into a threat in some way and lead to feelings of gloom. The least gesture of disapproval may bring about extremes of feeling, followed abruptly by a mood of the opposite end of the emotional spectrum. Such swings are not usually overwhelming, but these moods of optimism are all too often followed by ones of despair and pessimism before swinging back to feelings of hope, certainty and positive assurance.

Swift mood changes are common in adolescence and often intense. The basic problem is a variation on the theme of depressive tendencies with a veering away from depressive anxieties into a 'peak' excitable phase of over-activity and elation. Such swings can last anything from a few hours to days or weeks, but the personality invariably falls back into the depressive slide at some time. The over-active phase nearly always precedes the depression, sometimes quite subtly, and is the cause for much of the subsequent gloom and pessimism. Any chance happening, meeting or remark can rapidly worsen a mood because of the tendency to interpret negatively and personally whatever is said or done. This includes a most intense and undermining form of self-criticism, so that however the individual 'performs' or reacts to a situation, it is always felt to be inadequate and weak. In this respect they do not spare themselves, reflecting a marked tendency to masochism. A bout of high spirits always signals the crest of the wave and both follows and precedes a depressive mood. Sometimes a high follows an apparently quiescent and plateau period but shame, guilt and depression, related to imagined indiscretions during the highs, are never far away and seem to prevent a stable norm being attained.

In general, there is a lack of enthusiasm and energy for most things and often these individuals are their own worst enemy. At times the world seems a better, brighter and nicer place, filled with sympathetic people, out to help. This leads to sudden feelings of enthusiasm and optimism with drive and plans for the future; at the same time, contrasting feelings are always present to some degree, expressed as comments on 'the bloody-minded others', putting them 'in their place', or 'giving them something to think about'. Such outspoken aggressive statements do not of course endear them or lead to a position of stability or confidence as it is far too brittle.

Such swings are always a feature where insecurity is marked and the temperament unstable, unpredictable and emotionally labile. These problems affect the personal and emotional life of the individual and also the whole family. Mood swings are sudden and unpredictable; one outstanding feature is that often there is no obvious trigger to warn or account for the sudden changes. Living with a 'mood swinger' is like living on a knife edge or on a tight-rope. Because they are so sensitive, the least remark or comment can have an adverse effect and on most days something has been said to offend or upset.

Only rarely is there an optimistic or positive viewpoint. When this does happen, all too often it is based on assumption or distortion and doomed to disappointment. Their expectations are far too high to be realizable and, living on the fringe of reality, often in a vacuum, much of the time, they have no real ideas as to how others see or experience them. Only in the 'high' phase are they ever actively involved and more at the centre of things, otherwise they live near to a phantasy world; not that this world of assumption and imagination stops them reacting to what they think was intended. In the high of the mood swing, certainty and knowing is at a peak and can easily lead to a blow-out of feelings and overreactions. This can place additional pressure on friends and family, making living with such individuls a matter of greater uncertainty and chance. However, they are never boring at such times and each day brings its fill of drama and action — unfortunately, around the insensitivities of others. Insight into their own lack of awareness and self-centredness is painfully lacking, especially during the excitable moods.

Because of these long-standing mood swings, planning can be difficult and dominated by a desire for change — as is reflected in the aims and ambitions of these personalities. There is a desire to 'change the world' but at the same time they feel frustrated and unable to realize such lofty aims so that, as a result, all ambition at a more mundane level is abandoned. These ideals are a reflection of inner psychological patterns and imagery of the world as they see it. The swings reflect instability of personality and the ideals can all too quickly give way to moods of defeatism, withdrawal, lack of confidence and motivation. There is so much that they could and would do 'if only' — others would listen and heed them. At such times they feel that they have the 'answers'. Unfortunately, such periods or solutions are not built upon bricks of reality or reality-perceptions and such misconceived windmills rarely gain much credence from the family who know them over the years.

During the highs there is constant gaiety and hilarity, the individual is seen as apparently outgoing, forceful and confident, although at times insistent and dominating to the point of being irritating. Any telephone in their vacinity is irresistable and used for lengthy calls to ring up one friend after the other. The drive to have friends is a powerful one and reflects a basic need of reassurance. Expensive gifts or visits, overspending on clothes or speculative buying from a stockbroker can all lead to a trail of disaster when the bills come in and friends are no longer interested or available. Borrowing from these newly acquired friends — debts very rarely repaid — leads to rapid alienation and the urgent need to find others to 'fill the gap' during the next high.

Because of personal instability, these characters tend to be very unreliable and particularly unsound in business — taking risks, chances and often short-cuts which can be both costly and disastrous. All too often they shift from over-cautious hesitancy and backing down to making rash decisions without consulting with their partners. The mood swings are always worse in women at period times and often directly related to them because of the hormonal imbalance — although this is not the root cause of their problem but only an added stress.

Some Causative Factors of Mood Swings

The background of these personalities is usually an urban one, often with an absent or working mother or a split or second marriage, occurring during the key early years or adolescence or immediately before in late childhood. Usually there have been problems with a brother or sister, which were not resolved by the family or acknowledged. In others, the sibling gap was over four years and could not be bridged to form a closeness between them. There were often marked phantasies of rage and jealousy concerning a brother or sister in childhood, but there were never admitted or shown, the feeling being that the other was older, more successful, more favoured by the parents and that they themselves were not really listened to or valued as much in terms of their own ideas and wishes.

Recommended Remedies for Mood Swings

1) *Apis*
This is indicated for restless excitability, where there is a need of company and periods of hysterical depression. In general they are thirstless, resembling *Pulsatilla* characteristics in this respect. Often little water is passed and there is a tendency to jealousy. At times they swing to a mood of agitation, convinced that they are about to die, and in general there is little that is quiet, peaceful or restful in their make-up.

2) *Arsenicum*
As time passes so slowly, these personalities are always in a hurry and usually restless and exasperated, easily swinging from fear and anxiety to excitement or irritability. In general, they need company and people, fearing being left alone. Often they are very weak, apathetic and exhausted, quite unable to think clearly or concentrate to find the word or phrase that escapes them. This makes for many gaps in their memory and in their thinking. Fear of failure makes for many of their impulsive attitudes and mood swings.

3) *Calcarea*
This remedy is indicated in cases of weakness, depression and chilliness, when the individual is full of restless fears and twitches, and at other times critical of others, restless, impatient or excitable. The apathy, weakness and marked dampness of the head and forehead from sweating is the most marked feature.

4) *Natrum mur.*
This remedy is indicated when the individual is highly nervous with bouts of hysterical behaviour or hypochondriacal preoccupations. The mood varies from one of almost an exalted high with laughter to one of tears, depression and gloom. They are often depressed, preferring their own company to that of others and in particular to any form of

consolation. Constipation is common and reflects their need to keep everything under control and suppressed until tension overspills as a mood swing.

5) *Nux vomica*
This is the great remedy for contrasts of mood, in particular spasmodic contrasts. There is a powerful need of solitude and withdrawal in these individuals, as well as the overpowering impulse to speak their mind and to say what they think — whatever the costs. This often contributes to their fits of depression, anxiety and moody doubts. Periods of excitement and agitation can also occur, but are always spasmodic, short-lived, and often with poor controls.

6) *Phosphorus*
There are flashes of sudden anger or change of mood which varies from anxiety or fear to anger, the need of attention with laughter and a sudden high phase. But these personalities are not stable in any of their moods, quickly becoming irritable, volatile, sometimes to the point of delusional beliefs. The chest or liver and gall-bladder are particularly vulnerable areas for them physically and are rarely absent as complaints in one form or other.

7) *Pulsatilla*
This is the great remedy associated with variation and change. The basic physique and temperamental make-up must fit the remedy. Change at all levels is characteristic so that these people can at times be typically yielding and compliant yet flare up into a rage and ill humour when criticized, then burst into floods of tears until these are replaced by sudden smiles when the audience is sufficiently controlled and subdued. They are quickly and frequently depressed, however, as lack of confidence is their great weakness and this makes them too easily influenced by others. Often everything is either idealized or seems beyond them. They are like the wind flower, constantly changing, dependent upon others to an extreme degree and over-reacting to external events and pressures. All of this makes them extremely vulnerable and malleable and contributes largely to their underlying misery and lack of satisfaction.

Manic-depressive Illness
This is a more serious form of illness with severe mood disturbance and complete loss of any sense of reality. It is commonly seen in adults of the 40-50 year age group, more rarely in younger people. There is a

severe recurrent condition, present over many months or years, the onset obscure, although sometimes following a disastrous marital break-down, redundency threat or loss of job. Frequently, the personality make-up of the individual is of phobic or obsessional tendency. Sometimes there has been the loss of a close member of the family and the grief has been too much to bear without break-down and a flight into manic-depressive confusion.

There have been other cases that I have known where a heavy financial loss has occurred in the area of business which the individual is responsible for. The loss may not necessarily have been of his making, but nevertheless he blames himself severely for it. The basic personality is partly at fault — they are always very reliable, conscientious, hard-working to a fault, but of rigid and perfectionist temperament, double checking and too controlled and orderly in most things. There is also a tendency to mood swings over the years, not necessarily in a severe form until the acute illness takes over.

The precipitating cause is nearly always an acute shock or trauma of some kind which tips the balance from mood swings into the more severe psychosis. There is a constant need of success in everything in order to boost the deflated ego, weakened by periods of depression and self-criticism, and such personalities often attempt to prove themselves in business fields. As they are so dedicated and hard-working, often highly successful in terms of work output, they tend to do particularly well in this field. However, they also take risks and this makes them vulnerable. When a plan goes wrong, there is inevitably the feeling of depression and discouragement in spite of the fact that it was no fault of their own. They have the frequent morbid tendency to feel personally responsible for the ills of the world which sit uncomfortably on their shoulders, and when things go wrong or not according to plan, they make themselves ill by worrying unduly so that it is often at this point that the manic-depressive cycle starts up. At such times they become like an engine out-of-phase, taking on a new and more highly pitched, uncontrollable rhythm with its own rules and patterns.

There is always a break with reality; the high hypomanic episodes are usually periods of extreme activity, excessive talking, laughter, over-activity and delusional beliefs, often of a persecutory nature. These beliefs commonly relate to a recent event, trauma or illness. They feel themselves to be the centre of attention, involved internationally with the F.B.I. or the secret service. Such delusional systems often contain an important household name, sometimes known to them in reality from business contacts, although others are usually pure phantasy. Such figures are usually felt to be spreading malicious and damaging rumours about them. These delusional, paranoid beliefs are a common feature of manic-depression and represent one of its more serious aspects because this psychotic component undermines judgement, thinking and perception. In many ways the delusional beliefs resemble a schizophrenic illness, although the overall outlook and prognosis is less severe. There is, however, the same inability to differentiate phantasy from reality, leading to a delusional, confused state of mind and the utmost conviction as to the reality of the beliefs. In order to explain the frequent lethargy and depression, they develop explanations based on the belief that they are being interfered with and drugged. For instance, they believe L.S.D. is being piped into their home in an extraordinary fashion — through the letter box or gas taps, in order to undermine and control them. The 'persecutors' are nearly always success stories in some way or in the news, at the top of their profession — hence their preoccupation and phantasy-involvement with them — and this, combined with the constant name-dropping, helps to combat the feelings of underlying inadequacy and hopelessness at their situation.

Although most of the time they are convinced of the reality of their delusional beliefs, at other times there are flashes of insight, but these are usually too short-lasting to help them with the severity of the mental state.

Because of their drive, enthusiasm and apparent confidence, particularly during a 'high' period, their work output has often been phenomenal and for many years they may have been able to cover up their periods of inactivity and depression. Because of their drive and successful track record, there are a wide variety of influential and successful friends and colleagues, admiring their tremendous verve, output and energy. In addition, they also have a positive flair for business and until judgement breaks down, for long periods, their professional results are often startling and impressive. Because of these contacts and their business background, it is not always easy to differentiate reality from gross delusion, at least not initially, until unreality sets in. However optimistic, energetic and over-active they may have been during a manic phase, contrasting feelings of defeat and depression are never further than just around the corner. In the same way, these types are never very far away from a 'high' either, because of the constant flight from depression.

For many years, a 'high' has been the norm, with little need for sleep, endless energy and rarely tired since they blossom at night, taking on more and more with seeming confidence and no apparent difficuly. Much of their success is to impress others and to bolster their very low self-estem. Eventually all of this takes its toll with exhaustion, insomnia and weakness. As soon as the energy surge is over — then the depression sets in, as physically they are just not able to continue the acute phase of activity. There may have been several attempts at suicide, some of them serious. During this acute phase they may be unable to work because of the degree of exhaustion, weakness and delusional process, all of which combine to undermine health and judgement. In general, there is a strong drive to work, in order to prove themselves capable of succeeding in the major area where they have flair and ability. Their chronic insomnia is often aggravated by anti-depressants and tranquillizers that they may be taking, often adding to their fatigue and depression.

Plausibility makes manic-depressives as much a danger to themselves as to others because of their intelligence, ability to communicate verbally, and likeable, confident manner. This image may last for many months or years and only begins to crumble when their conduct becomes increasingly bizarre and repetitive. Complaints of unfair treatment, lack of sympathy and understanding are numerous, often put down initially to stress. Usually there is no lasting insight present and they are quite convinced that these beliefs are valid. Doubts expressed by others are seen as part of the plot to discredit them, alienate, and ultimately to destroy them. This overwhelming conviction of persecutory threats with no understanding of their distorted perceptions and the extent of the self-damage, is a danger to the whole integrity and health of the personality and sanity, reflecting the very serious nature of the illness.

Recommended Remedies for Manic-depression

Because of the severe nature of manic-depressive psychosis' it is not considered suitable for teatment by the family except under the direction of a physician.

1) *Agaricus*

There are extremes of mood and excitement with phantasies of grandeur or power conflicting with further periods of severe depression and suicidal intentions. Nervous muscular twitchings are marked as well as a very poor peripheral circulation — the hands and feet often blue with cold.

2) *Anacardium orientale*

There is an over-active state with loss of control, swearing, irritability, or a dream-like state with marked delusions. There is a danger of suicide by shooting.

3) *Medorrhinum*

There is a deluded, restless, depressive state. These patients are full of doom and gloom and fearful at all times; at other periods, they are impatient and always in a hurry as time is experienced as passing too slowly. Absolute certainty of beliefs and convictions is a marked feature.

4) *Platina*

The mental state is usually profoundly disturbed with severe confusion and the characteristic tendency to look down on others and to feel elevated and proud. They are often very irritable to an extreme degree and violent at times because of their confusion. In a manic phase they are full of their own self-importance, and the deep sense of emptiness only occurs in the down phase, although it is never far away really from their fragile elevated state of superiority.

When the psychotic phase is severe their body image becomes fragmented and their arm or limbs are not felt to be attached to their body or indeed to belong to them.

5) *Lachesis*

There is a restless, nervous exitement where jealousy, suspicion and a preoccupation with others is marked. The mood is very variable and in general the person feels controlled and influenced by others because of their suspicions and doubts about others — really about themselves at a deeper level. The mood may be severely agitated and hypermanic when there is a tendency to mock and satirize others. Talking is a problem as they will never stop unless completely exhausted. Intolerence of tight clothing is another important feature. Aggravation through sleep is the major unusual diagnostic feature so that they wake from sleep at any time, unrefreshed and more agitated.

6) *Aconitum*

This remedy is of value in the very acute cases in those personalities of plethoric build, strong and muscular with a history of many acute fears of phases of excitability.

7) *Belladonna*

There is an acute manic-depressive condition with a restless, suicidal, depressive mood, swinging abruptly into mania — dancing, laughing, shouting and confused so that control is difficult. Violence is often a feature, especially when thwarted. In all cases where the remedy is accurately indicated, there is a combination of burning heat and redness, often of the face. The least touch, draught or jar always characteristically worsens the condition, and aggravates the mental state.

15.

OBSESSIONAL STATES AND HYPOCHONDRIASIS

Everyone, to some extent, has a susceptibility to obsessional behaviour in their make-up. Even when temporary, it is always a reflection of underlying insecurity, whatever the reasons, and it may be seen from the childhood onwards. In the child it is usually shown by a meticulous control and neatness, especially at play, and in a very precise arrangement and movement of toys or games. Most children are naturally untidy, obviously varying with the individual, but a scrupulous concern for detail and order at the expense of more creative and adventurous play is not usual unless there is marked obsessional anxiety. An excessive degree of arrangement and rearrangement is strongly indicative of obsessional thinking, where all play, movement and activity is suddenly suspended. In others, obsessional fear can lead to isolation, making it difficult to clearly define the underlying nature of the problem. Elective mutism is an example of this. The child is totally mute, withdrawn and obsessional, remote from everyone except the mother, seeming to communicate with her only from fear of being abandoned or annihialated.

In many cases, both pot-training and upbringing has been over-emphasized from a very early age and has been a preoccupation of the mother or grandparents. Strict demands may have been imposed for cleanliness and control. The pressures — a clear condition for love and acceptance have meant that the child is obediently clean and scrupulously dry at an excessively early age, the infant potted for long periods in some cases to ensure this. Often there is a combination of strict bowel training by a family which has a long history of such bowel problems as colitis, constipation or diverticulitis where making a mess and the fear of soiling has become a preoccupation of the adults involved in the child's upbringing. Such excessive concerns by the family can clearly undermine all confidence and flexibility in the developing infant. For the sake of cleanliness and order there is interference with all the normal phases of personality growth and maturation, engendering deep-seated fears, anxiety and resentment which are commonly at the roots of the obsessional problem.

When there is this family tendency to bowel problems together with such early pressures upon the developing personality, the stage is set for a later obsessional disorder.

In the adult, obsessional states are always a form of excessive control in a rigid type of personality make-up. Much of the stiffness and stuffy rigidity is inherited and the same traits can be seen in other members of the close family. Threatened by change in any form whatsoever, they are overwhelmed by the fears of anything different or new. All their energies and personality defences are directed at preserving the familiar so that, psychologically, they can remain safe and usually inert. Such patterns may also be seen in any institutional establishment where both individuals and organizing staff give priority to no change and non-interference. The aim is a minimum of disturbance in any form to ensure a reassuring continuity. This makes for continual warding-off of any attempts at modernization or change and in most cases this is felt to be outside interference. Change in any form, however detailed, small or trivial is always unwelcome because it is felt to be such a threat and it can quickly become a source of anxiety and panic.

The obsessive personality always tends to make others wait for him, needing to be in control whatever the situation; without this they easily go to pieces. At certain times anything is seen as a threat and leads to argument, reproaches and irritability. An open window becomes a source of violent danger and an emotional outburst may follow, because of the possibility of dust, broken glass or insects getting into the food and poisoning them. Everything must be checked and double checked out of doubt and fear of making a mistake or missing something. This lack of confidence in their own judgement means that doors, taps, locks and switches are constantly re-checked, using up valuable time, delaying and holding up the work of the day. Above all else they seek to avoid the present and the future because of these overwhelming threats of growth and change.

For the obsessional type, all life and occurrences — the least noise, request, letter or telephone call is beset with potential danger which threatens security. Appointments, bills and travel are all put off for as long as possible or, paradoxically, attended to prematurely in an attempt to control fate and 'get in first'. Being life's pessimists, they see themselves as living in a world full of danger, dominated by the constant threat of malice or bad luck. They spend their lives dominated by their phantasies, on the defensive against every aspect of living, repeating charms and recipes for safety in one form or another as an expression of their superstitious thinking.

At all times there is a profound sense of being just one step away from disaster so that involvement, contact with others, or any form of movement or indeed of life tends to be protective. It is generally believed and expected that at any moment some happening will change their precarious comfort and security for the worst. The typical outlook is always one of impending disaster and even a positive event, good news, or good luck is only cautiously and slowly admitted to.

Usually the obsessed character will deny any controlling or aggressive features, although this is seen clearly in the way they make their friends the victims of their neurosis. They remain unaware of the damage they can inflict upon those involved with them by their obsessions, controlling ways and fears. Feeling defenseless against life's injustices, they spend their time in a running battle with life, warding off fate by their own particular brand of magic and ritual and a form of thinking that ensures rigidity and immobility at all levels. Their lives are dominated by attempts to stave off the blows of an angry god, full of disapproval and punishment for their omissions, but they fail to see how such a god reflects their own infantile feelings of rage and resentment.

The obsessional mind is one which in many ways has progressed little from one of the primitive omnipotence of the young child. It retains all the limitations and drawbacks of thinking based on emotional conviction and knowing with absolute certainty. Such certainty-beyond-doubt also contributes to the usually marked features of control — both of others as well as of themselves. They quite naturally assume that they are threatened by the dictates of an all-powerful fate and in every obsessional state this emphasis on 'control' is usually predominant. Such problems can often be linked to early toilet-training and pressures which in many cases have been either unduly severe or insensitive to the developing child's individual needs; the strictness of such an attitude may have contributed to a failure to mature emotionally and a persistence of early infantile attitudes and assumptions, carried over into the adult mind.

Rigidity is seen in the physical poise and movement which is often ungainly, but especially it is seen in the typical mental attitudes. Strictly conformist, they always go by the book and any request for modification of established patterns is delayed or thought about so deeply as to all possible ramifications and implications, in the hope that if only they can sit and wait long enough the demand will go away.

Sitting on things for as long as possible has always been an obsessional characteristic. Alternatively, decisions are referred to a superior so that nothing need be done at present and the evil day is put off until later or held at a safer distance from the present. The obsessional mind is well fitted for the role of life's civil servant, living a red-tape restrictive life in every thought, word and deed. Whenever possible they avoid taking any responsibilities or decisions and in some ways are ideally suited for service life where all decisions can be referred and no individual initiative or commitment need ever be taken. They lack, however the initiative required for the commissioned ranks and a position of real authority or responsibility for others.

New ideas are opposed on principle and are rarely given serious consideration. A request for anything at all unusual is treated by a blank refusal and often amazement. The obsessive character is intellectual and sees the pitfalls of change clearly and logically, but never the advantages. When serving on a committee, they can be relied upon to strongly oppose attempts at modernization and are always supporters of the establishment and the status quo.

'Magical thinking' is the key to understanding the obsessional personality and such thinking is nearly always highly secretive and rarely talked about because it is felt to be so very powerful. Yet it is a dominating feature and plays a major role in their lives. The thought processes come quite close to the delusional at times and only differ from it because there is no real break with the world of reality, unless the illness has proceded to a schizophrenic one. Obsessional thinking is highly organized, remote from feelings and sensitivity and centred around theoretical speculation and the boundless possibilities of the imagination.

Dependence is a marked feature in their make-up, together with a profound sense of vulnerability. All self-dependency and growth of confidence is suspended by the personality weakness and vulnerability, since the obsessional patterns and fixations prevent the important building up of a broad and deep range of life's experiences.

In most cases, the worst fear is the loss of a much-needed key person who must often remain nameless, but whom the obsessional feels totally dependent upon psychologically for survival. The ultimate fear is the unspeakable one — namely the loss of this person by accident, death or illness. A patient, one of twins, contacted chicken pox at an early age and 'gave' the illness to her twin sister. Unfortunately, the illness took a much more severe form in the twin, with complications leading to meningitis and a fatal outcome. Since that time the patient has feared destroying anyone at all closely involved with her and dreaded being responsible for a repetition of the earlier tragedy, particularly to someone most needed. The natural infantile ambivalence was in this case most strongly reinforced by the very real loss of the sister and this had dominated her life and thinking since that time. In all relationships there is an ambivalence, and between twins, however close, it is also present so that problems of envy, rivalry and jealousy arise at some time as part of the contrasts of life and living. Usually it is 'worked through', or to come to terms with by the bonds of closeness and affection unless, as with the patient described, the caring, reparative phase of ambivalence is interfered with by illness or loss.

The obsessional fears the consequences of his own ambivalence acting in some uncontrolled way and alienating him from essential contacts and closeness. This is a very powerful feature of the whole illness. It is almost as if some inconsequential and insignificant action will suddenly bring about irretrievable loss. Such feelings, although largely unconscious, are only just under the surface and the feared catastrophe is always one which threatens to leave them helpless and without support.

The whole adventure of life is a thing which is avoided because of the overwhelming fear of letting go. For the obsessional personality, challenge, the whole chain of life's events is not one of excitement, anticipation, pleasure and wonder, but rather an experience of peril to be avoided at all costs. Living is felt only in terms of extremes, without pleasure. Only the worst is ever expected, and this is their reason for constantly attempting to control and to crush life before they themselves are crushed by it.

Locked into his defences, this personality is the victim of his own cautionary measures. At all times he fears losing control, especially of the ambivalent aggressiveness and violence, although its existence is totally denied by his apparent masochism and passivity. Such denial causes them to feel that their suppressed aggression has a life of its own which constantly boomerangs back at them, threatening them and their loved ones. Much of the aggression is because of unconscious resentment towards these loved and needed ones because they are so special and therefore a potential cause of vulnerability. The whole problem of need and vulnerability is reinforced by parental rigidity and interference during the early toilet training period, or by any psychological loss or trauma happening at this time which can be later attributed to their own omnipotence.

The Homoeopathic Contribution to Obsessional Disease
If we now consider the homoeopathic remedies, how they work and the level at which they have influence upon the mental processes, we can

begin to see why they can be effective in what is a seemingly intractable and chronic disease.

The homoeopathic remedies act by loosening up and lessening rigidity of personality so that more movement and flexibility of attitude is possible. The perceptions of and attitudes towards others are generally widened and improved. Homoeopathy can open up closed and sealed areas of tissues, but it also acts in a similar way on walled up areas of the mind, enabling more contact at an emotional level as there is less defensiveness and fewer assumptions about other people's motivations with a more realistic appraisal of others.

Because homoeopathy acts so deeply, especially in the higher potencies, it relaxes the patient and reduces fearfulness, panic and anxiety. The remedies, when accurately prescribed, have the power to lessen the extent of distorted perspectives of an unhealthy kind. As the external threats and fears are reduced, so the defensive obsessional formulae can also be reduced overall and limited to more acceptable and controllable limits.

Because the remedies give a real relief from symptoms, this allows the possibility of a more positive and concentrated approach in the work areas, and a lessening of the patient underselling and undervaluing himself. Promotion and the beginning of some real achievement is possible once new and real confidence can be engendered as the obsessional process is put more into perspective.

The remedies can act in some cases very quickly, lessening and breaking down obsessional patterns present for many years. They facilitate or loosen up or ease relationships, so that the patient can make more mature contact with others at a realistic level, rather than only in terms of obsessional phantasies and fears about their motivations. Such reality-based contacts have far more stability and satisfaction when there is real contact and a real sharing and beginning of trust can be established.

The well prescribed remedy not only relaxes the patient physically, but by relaxing cramps and spasms due to tension, it builds up confidence and relieves frequent hypochondriacal tendencies commonly due to interpreting everything that happens or is felt in a negative way.

The remedy must be given in a high dilution or potency to be effective, and should be repeated as soon as the symptoms show any signs of returning because of the chronic and deep-seated nature of the psychological problem. Also, the action of the remedies has a limited life of weeks, varying with the particular remedy used.

A combination of homoeopathic remedies and explorative consultations is usually needed to allow the underlying fears and doubts to come to the surface — and this may take several weeks or months to complete. In some cases there is a very rapid relief and improvement. More often it is slow because of the number of years that the problem has been present.

Part of the difficulty to be breached in treating the obsessional is the very profound opposition by the ill part of the patient to curing himself and indeed to any form of change whatsoever, because it is felt to be an intrusion rather than a relief. In addition, treatment is often met with suspicion and resentment. Often, the obsessional with all the limitations and drawbacks of their illness nevertheless prefers their condition to one of change to health and ultimately of challenge.

Recommended Remedies for Obsessional States

1) *Aurum met.*
There is a depressive obsessional disorder and a preoccupation with death and dying. Suicidal thoughts are often present, the mind ruminates over ways of ending it all and suicidal phantasies to the exclusion of all else. The other major area of obsessional thinking is centred around self-reproach, unworthiness generally, feelings of neglect and failure. These ideas take over everything and dominate every aspect of the personality, creating a suicidal risk. There may have been attempts to end life in the past. Difficulties of a physical nature, involving the heart, liver or joints with rheumatic problems are commonly present.

2) *Aconitum*
This is usually indicated for the more acute problem where fear and anxiety dominate all aspects of normal living. Especially, there is fear of death and of dying at a certain hour, which the individual is able to predict with supposed accuracy. There is also fear of the dark, of shadows, of crossing the street, and in the background of all this is anxiety without any real cause or basis, and without logic or real purpose. Restlessness and agitation are always typical features associated with this remedy.

3) *Anacardium*
There are many bizarre, obsessional ideas — a constant and worrying smell of burning wood or smoke. The individual is feeble-minded, weak and exhausted, unable to concentrate or to remember clearly, often irritable or contradictory. The weakness of recall is compensated for and hidden by the common tendency for heavy swearing which is often

repetitive and obsessional. The personality dissociation creates an illness that borders on the psychotic at times.

4) *Hyoscyamus*
There is a depressed obsessional state with periods of irritability and excitement, often with a marked phobic element present, particularly a fear of being left alone in the house, of being bitten by a dog or poisoned, so that all food, medicine and any form of treatment is regarded with the utmost suspicion and mistrust. There is also a characteristic fear of water, especially of drowning. Obsessional counting is also a feature (compare *Calcarea*), or there is a preoccupation with frequent hand-washing — the hands often feel strange, at times too large. Another feature is the compulsive arrangement of all objects into controlled lines and patterns on wallpaper or elsewhere. When in a severely excitable state, they can become deluded to the point of seeing long lines of insects, also in patterns.

5) *Cicuta*
There is a tendency to rigid, obsessional thinking, with marked anxiety and fears. Confusion and suspicion are also marked. This remedy is of value in difficult, chronic cases, particularly where there is a history of fits and convulsions or epilepsy in the family or as part of the mental pattern.

6) *Cuprum met.*
There is a fearful, anxious state of mind, with many restless, uneasy, compulsive patterns of behaviour and tremblings with the intensity of the feelings and involvement. Spasms and muscular cramps are always present to some degree so that twichings and jerky movements are common. There are often bouts of obsessional behaviour, the mood taking over the whole body as well as the mind; and then suddenly the mood is over.

7) *Belladonna*
This is recommended for the acute attacks of more violent and active obsessional states with fixed, rigid ideas and tendencies towards anger, impatience, even violence when there is any form of opposition or disagreement. Heat and redness are nearly always present, with a flushed, hot and anxious face as the intensity of the obsession mounts.

8) *Ignatia*

Irritable and full of changeable contradictions, there is complete lack of confidence in these characters with much double checking of doors and switches. Often tearful, they are always worse for any form or fright or emotion. At times they are quiet and withdrawn and are unable to get a person or a thought out of their mind. Any feelings of anger, regret, resentment or disappointment are completely denied and buried in the depths of the mind, reinforcing the obsessional tendencies because all feelings are suppressed. This denial also promotes the common tendency to hysterical behaviour.

9) *Lachesis*

There are many obsessional fears and sexual preoccupations, centred around feelings of jealousy and suspicion. They often feel that others are criticizing them so that they are often on the defensive. Exhaustion is marked, with an aggravation on waking or after sleep when the general state of nervousness and obsessional thinking and fears are worse. There is intolerance of tight clothing of any sort. In general, this is a basically self-destructive personality with marked lack of confidence, self-doubts and depression. The feelings of depression can be severe, with an extreme degree of self-criticism and irritability. They reproach themselves severely and there seems, at times, no way of stopping such negative behaviour. At other times the accusations and betrayal are turned on another victim as part of the conviction of jealousy or suspicion and mistrust. There is a lot of barely covered aggression which all too easily comes to the surface, making them difficult to live or work with.

10) *Stramonium*

This is a remedy for the most disturbed states with terrifying obsessional thought on the border-line of delusional thought. The images provoke restlessness and excitement, easily leading to violence at times. At other times there is complete withdrawal and mutism.

11) *Silicea*

This remedy is indicated for long-standing, chronic obsessional states where weakness and exhaustion are marked. Depression and irritability are also common features, expressing feelings of futility and of lack of strength. In general, there is a preoccupation with failure and a pronounced fear of others. Embarrassed and over-sensitive to an extreme degree, these individuals are dominated by fear, weakness and fixed ideas of impotence, or of any public talk or engagement that they must make. There is an obsessional conviction of their own inadequacy which can be quite paralyzing, and at times, in despair, they can spend hours obsessively counting small objects as buttons or pins.

12) *Pulsatilla*

I have found this to be one of the major remedies for obsessional disease when the underlying physical traits and personality match the remedy. It can be very helpful, even in long-standing, chronic cases, and can break the pattern of obsessional thinking when all other treatments have failed, the change taking place rapidly. The remedy must be repeated as soon as the symptoms show any sign of returning, but not before, at the risk of re-establishing the disease patterns.

13) *Thuja*

Depressive obsessional anxiety is the main problem here, with many bizarre, fixed ideas of an obsessional nature which cannot be alleviated by reason or reassurance. Strangeness of phantasy and ideas is marked, so that, for instance, they experience a live animal in the abdomen, or feel that body and soul are separated, the body made of brittle glass that will break at any moment. In the elderly obsessional, the typical headaches occur, very localized, as if a nail is being driven through the skull or like an isolated piece of lead in just one small area and these are often relieved by this remedy when all other attempts have only served to worsen the condition.

14) *Veratrum alb.*

This is of value in the obsessional illness of the puerperal type (following childbirth). There is depression, a pale appearance, and an obsessional desire to tear, cut or to destroy, which is compulsive and very disturbing.

15) *Cannabis indica*

This is indicated where there is an excitable obsessional state with fixed ideas and remoteness from reality. Time passes all too slowly, so that they are forgetful, dissociated, seem elsewhere and preoccupied. There is a great fear of death or of madness and of being locked away. Thoughts and ideas rush through the mind, often unfinished, confused and uncertain, then returning to their fixed obsessional pattern.

16) *Sulphur*

This is a useful remedy for chronic long-standing cases, especially where there is intolerance of heat and an untidy mind, full of speculations, fears and weakness. Marked anxiety is a typical feature and the skin is usually chronically infected and re-infected by the compulsive picking and touching which is another feature of the remedy-picture.

16.

PSYCHOSEXUAL PROBLEMS

As with adult personality and adult confidence, adult sexuality also takes its origins from the child's earliest experiences and security and is inseparable from it. The sense of security and identification is clearly seen in the young child's games and play. During these key formative years, there is a giving out of mutual caring, closeness and sharing by both child and parents, which gives the foundation to all later tenderness, sensuality and security.

Without exception, the psychology of each adult is rooted in the quality of infantile development and such infantile aspects are never far removed from adult tenderness and mature, caring relationships. In the early fore-play of adult sexuality, such infantile roots can be clearly expressed and exchanged between the partners, but does not play a dominant role in the whole sexual experience. When there is an excessive attachment to the infantile roots of development, this can distort the adult sexual relationship into a narcissistic experience which emerges as a perversion; for example the need for indecent exposure and voyeurism. What should be a mutual and intimate sharing of affection and loving becomes a fleeting, compulsive and often aggressive act which involves the other as a distant phantasy object rather than as a person to be cared for and appreciated in his own right.

Masturbation

Until relatively recently masturbation was given pride of place, or rather blame, as the basic and most frequent cause of ill health and, without question, the root of all mental illness. Most Victorian medical textbooks were quite obsessed with onanism as a major social evil and the practise was exposed and moralized about with all the fervour of a witch-hunt or inquisition. Not surprisingly, this preoccupation by the physicians of the day was no more than a reflection of society generally — both towards masturbation and sexuality generally. Much of the prevailing guilt, confusion and shame ended up as an untwinable knot in the psyche of the adolescent of the day, who felt as if each act was a repetition of original sin leading to damnation and madness.

As every parent and adult knows, masturbation occurs openly and naturally in all children from their earliest age and is a feature of normal infantile curiosity and exploration of themselves and those close to them. It is also a marked feature of normal adolescence, indicating a resurgence of infantile aspects, as well as hormonal levels reaching a peak in the mid-teens and stimulating libido to a maximum. Masturbation is now not normally a problem for many people; indeed it is an act of release and pleasure. When there is a problem, it lies with the suppression of masturbation, particularly when guilt is associated, sometimes leading to an excessive compulsive continuation into adulthood.

Masturbation both expresses sexuality and gives it an outlet, with a relief from built up tensions, phantasies and excitements which it is impossible to otherwise express. Particularly in the adolescent there is a build up of sexual energies and phantasies which could be overwhelming without the release that masturbation provides quite naturally; as the adolescent matures physically and psychologically at an increasingly younger age. Although primarily considered to be an adolescent problem, masturbation can be clearly observed in the young baby as an expression of comfort and erections are frequently present from an early age, beginning in the first few months of life.

Masturbation provides a way of resolving unconscious sexual phantasy and guilt, helping to deal with some of the anxiety concerned with growing up and becoming part of an adult world. Often the problems are really those of the parents reflecting their own repressive upbringing and unresolved guilts and pressures of their own background. Masturbation in children is quite normal, but a preoccupation with it is not, and reflects an immaturity of attitudes and a failure to intuitively comprehend the natural needs and developmental steps of the child. The combination of prudishness, purity, rigidity and control by the parents, together with attitudes which were not basically open, was typical of Victorian society, and destructive to the individual.

This unhealthy preoccupation of both the earlier physicians and the family at the turn of the century did much to instil an unhealthy sense of guilt and sexual repression in many families today. It still casts its shadow on freedom of expression, attitudes towards nudity and spontaneity, and it is only in recent years that it has been overcome. The present modern kick-back and trends in morality are very much a reaction to such unhealthy attitudes and repressions by teachers and parents, where over the years there was only a superficial show of concern for the needs and development of the child and adolescent.

When masturbation becomes excessive, obsessional or associated with excessively sadistic phantasies, it may then become a cause for concern. But this is the same for any aspect of the individual; eating or hand washing or dieting, if excessive or compulsive, is unhealthy and rooted in unreality and distortion, and therefore needing attention and help of some kind.

Recommended Remedies for Masturbation

Treatment should in all cases only be considered when masturbation is either excessive and obsessional, inappropriate or when painful. In all other occasions it is within normal experience, varying with the individual and a combination of hormonal and libidinal levels. In many cases the total lack of masturbation may be more abnormal then its healthy presence - indicative of undue rigidity or puritanism.

Excessive and Obsessional Masturbation

1) *Calcarea*

Indicated when the individual is pale, flabby and lacking in general stamina and energy. There is often a combination of agitation with anxiety and exhaustion. Often thoughts and ideas are turned round and round but no decisions are ever taken. Nothing really satisfies and whatever is eventually done is carried in a bored, exhausted way. Masturbation has often little to do with sexuality or libido, which is usually low, but is more of an automatic, compulsive act to release tension.

2) *Arsenicum*

Use this remedy for the person with similar chilliness to and the exhaustion of *Calcarea,* but when of firmer and much more compact build. It is often valuable when there is a severe and deep-seated obsessional make-up and where there is a combination of rigidity and ritual in many areas — masturbation being just one of them.

3) *Lachesis*

When the masturbation is reflecting a deep-seated personality disturbance, often with delusional features concerning sexual matters and almost an obsession with them. When this remedy is indicated there is also a disturbing area of suspicion and jealousy causing frequent problems and break-down of relationships. There is often a poor peripheral circulation giving a pallor and a waxy, bluish tint to the skin — reflecting the more generalized hormonal and circulatory disturbances which accompany the mental problems.

Inappropriate Masturbation

1) *Natrum mur.*
Usually there is a severe, sometimes chronic emotional problem with isolation and withdrawal, leading to disturbed and bizarre behaviour.

2) *Baryta carb.*
Compulsive, inappropriate masturbation may be an expression of senility or of sudden, degenerative, pre-senile changes when it occurs at a younger age. This remedy in the 30c potency is often helpful.

3) *Sulphur*
This remedy is indicated in cases of mental break-down and collapse of relationships so that behaviour and thinking has become a 'rag-bag' of bits and pieces of disjointed behaviour — nothing having any sense, except as a most isolated fragment of reality. Untidiness and disorder is common in every aspect of thinking, behaviour and appearance.

Painful Masturbation
The commonest causes are infective, mechanical or due to guilt. Any external mechanical factors such as adhesions, verruca or naevus, must be dealt with and rectified by the most appropriate treatment before commencing a homoeopathic approach to a possibly psychological cause.

1) *Nux vomica*
When pain is due to a combination of spasm and excessive tension, then in low 6c potency this remedy is often of value.

2) *Thuja*
I would recommend *Thuja* in the 30c potency for pain not due to physical causes, but where the cause is obscure or hidden, the attitudes rigid.

3) *Medorrhinum*
Use when there is any history of previous nfection, especially gonorrhoea, and where the pain seems to be occurring in the urethral area from spasm.

Homosexuality

A homosexual orientation is not in itself any form of sickness or illness. Inevitably it must be a sterile relationship as far as any experience of family is concerned.

Homosexuality has always existed and is common to both sexes. For the majority there are many unresolved problems and stereotyped assumptions and distortions of the opposite sex, which cause major difficulties, unless it is a friendly tolerance as sometimes exists between lesbian and homosexual. Usually there is a combination of competition and denigration involving the other sex, which does not occur to the same extent in the heterosexual couple. There is also considerable rivalry between heterosexual partners, so that often such relationships as are formed tend to be short-lasting, neurotic and unstable, and depression is common.

In many cases of male homosexuality there has been a severe trauma in the early formative years, affecting and distorting the whole sexual orientation — sometimes the loss of a parent at a key impressionable age, or an excessive close link with a parent, often an excessively clinging and hysterically possessive mother, preventing the real emergence of masculinity and independence. Sometimes such possessive relationships may continue well into middle age to the detriment of individual achievement and growth.

Some achieve a stable relationship and set up home together, forming a lasting bond which may last for many years, and this has become increasingly common for many homosexual men and women. Such couples are the fortunate ones and in many ways the exceptions. There are many who live lonely, isolated, 'closet' lives, sad and loveless, seemingly without aims or reason other than their work. Those that are fortunate enough to achieve a stable relationship have nevertheless all the problems of a heterosexual partnership without the bonus and joy of children.

For many, the homosexual orientation is not a total one, and it is common to find a bisexual attraction to the opposite sex which has never been allowed to expand and develop, but which emerges nevertheless in dreams or occasional impulses and phantasies. For some this poses a threat and such drives are quickly denied and suppressed. Others are able to express and to experience such opposing drives quite openly although they are usually lacking in depth.

In either male or female homosexuality, there is a division between the 'butch' or more masculine expression, and an effeminate one. It is not uncommon for there to be considerable antipathy, even violence, to occur between the two extremes and, like the anti-Semitic Jew, there is a form of violent 'butch' homosexual that cannot in any form tolerate effeminate queerness. Homosexuals as a group can be aggressive, but this is not the rule, and much more often they are the victims of aggression.

The main problem is not one of changing sexual orientation. Usually this has been established for many years, with the exception of some lesbian affairs started after the break-up of a marriage or affair, when it is not uncommon and indicative only of a temporary state of depression and loss of confidence. Such relationships are usually short-lasting and do not have the depth and commitment of the male homosexual attachment. A homosexual relationship may also sometimes occur in prison or in the services when there is deprivation of all female contact, but this kind is of only passing significance, and for the majority does not occur at all.

When help is needed it is often for problems of depression when a relationship has broken down, or for problems of tension, anxiety, promiscuity and futility. Hepatitis and venereal disease are complications of the common tendency to promiscuity, reflecting underlying instability and insecurity. But there is always need for attention, proof of being liked and lovable, hence the constant need to flirt, to gain attention, and to phantasize another conquest, another affair — however depressing, unsatisfactory and demoralizing. Without a continuing relationship homosexuality nearly always leads to a severe depressive problem, which needs urgent treatment.

With healthier, changing more accepting and mature attitudes towards homosexuality, there is now less need for gays to prove themselves in such clandestine ways as in the past, or for them to feel inferior citizens. Lesbian couples have always been far more accepted over the years, but it is only in recent years that the homosexual couple has been more accepted. The saddest cases are always those that have never declared not only their orientation, but themselves as people. They are the people of the shadows, and like peeping toms, or obscene telephone callers, live sad, sterile lives without purpose or caring. They rarely come for treatment, their deep-seated insecurities are such that they lack the insight to know that they have a problem that could be approached to find some answers and resolution.

Recommended Remedies for Some Aspects of Homosexuality
There are of course no specific remedies to treat homosexuality as such, and it should be regarded as a variation of the broad variety of man's sexual pattern which has always existed. In itself it is not an illness or a sickness that needs treating. When there are problems, these must be

dealt with as is appropriate for each individual. Problems often arise because there is a great deal of frustration and unhappiness, feelings of failure and lack of fulfilment. Many homosexuals do not achieve any form of deep or lasting relationship, causing depression. Promiscuity is a common problem which often occurs when there is a state of hyperactivity and excessive excitement — but often as a defence against depression.

Recommended Remedies for Homosexual Depression

1) *Natrum mur.*
This remedy is particularly helpful for the type of person that finds it difficult to mix, make relationships, or 'come out' — declare their orientation — because they are so withdrawn, frightened and lacking in confidence. The isolation is a powerful factor in the depression.

2) *Aurum mur.*
This is a useful remedy when depression is much more severe and profound, with a desperate note to it rather than a hysterical one — it should be given in the 30c potency.

Recommended Remedies for Homosexual Promiscuity
Promiscuity is not the usual reason why help is requested — it is much more a facet of a general often rather dangerous over-active state which may involve excesses in many areas including eating, smoking, alcohol and drugs, as well as the more direct sexual activity.

1) *Nux vomica*
This is the most useful remedy to use initially. There is often a lot of barely suppressed anger and rage that is being 'acted out' — for one reason or another, not infrequently to punish a partner who is felt to have been lacking in care and sensitivity. Such people are often also excessively hard-working and self-driving, and deal with underlying loneliness and depression by any form of excess — either at work or at leisure. They generally demand high standards of themselves as well as their partners — hence the frequent disappointments.

2) *Natrum mur.*
This is the alternative remedy which may alleviate compulsive, often self-destructive behaviour and help to break a pattern and open the way to new insights. It is best used in high potencies of 200c.

Recommended Remedies for Homosexual Insecurity

Again there are no specific remedies, and each individual must be treated in his own right according to the prevailing problems of the time. The most useful general remedy is always the constitutional one in a high potency of at least 200c. If there is an existing relationship which has problems of doubt and insecurity, these must be discussed openly within the relationship. If the insecurity is such that it has prevented any commitment from ever occurring, then there is a basic personality problem that needs exploring with support and treatment. In such cases, the general list of remedies under the section on insecurity should be considered to find the most appropriate for the individual make-up and particular form of insecurity.

Impotence

This is defined as weakness or absence of erection during the sexual act. Because masculine potency is so closely tied to underlying psychological attitudes and make-up it is not uncommon for temporary problems to occur, particularly in a sensitive person, whenever there is stress or pressure of any kind that is not brought to the surface, discussed and shared between the couple. Severe problems reflect a deeper lack of confidence or the inability to share a problem and sometimes a lack of trust within the relationship.

Sometimes the problem is one of long duration and has occurred in other relationships, with the ability to achieve penetration never well established since adolecence, indicating a more deep psychological problem with women generally, often going back to a disturbed relationship with the mother — who is ultimately the root of the masculine potency and confidence.

In other cases the male is passing through a personal crisis with periods of depression, withdrawal and general lack of confidence in every area. There is a failure to relate, to share and be open in all areas, because the problem is not recognized; alternatively the ability to communicate and to make contact with deeper feelings has never been developed or encouraged.

When the impotence is recent and confined to one relationship, then there is every possibility that it can be resolved by a combination of open discussion within the couple, and the appropriate homoeupathic remedy. It is only when there is an insensitive, non-caring response to sexual failure that it can become chronic and lead to complete and total withdrawal — as a form of self-protection. Because the problem is so closely tied to intimate psychological expressions and feelings, either of the couple may be responsible, and just as the male may provoke a reaction of frigidity in the woman, so too can the woman provoke and bring about impotency in the male.

Recommended Remedies for Impotency

1) *Lycopodium*
This remedy is particularly for the male that analyzes and thinks too much, so that everything is already anticipated, experienced and turned into a disaster before it has happened — the worst is always feared. Almost everything is turned into a performance and a test — in this case of virility — so that nothing is allowed to flow, be relaxed and enjoyed for the moment.

2) *Silicea*
This is useful in the low 6c potency whenever there is anxiety about fatigue, and general problems of exhaustion and lack of drive are prevalent.

3) *Calcarea*
This is best given in the 200c potency for the obese, flabby physique that is cold, has no energy, no real interest and drive, yet is tense and cannot relax.

4) *Arsenicum*
This is a similar remedy for weakness, but the physical make-up is different. If anything these individuals are too thin, too taught and tense, cannot relax and are always worried, fidgety, and obsessional. The over-active mind and body depletes them of all libido. Give in the 200c potency.

5) *Kali. carb.*
Weakness, fear, and dependency on the partner is the pattern here. These individuals cannot be alone, are full of fears and lacking in confidence, including in the libidinal sphere. Use the 200c potency.

6) *Nux moschata*
Use this remedy only when severe exhaustion is present to such a degree that every facet of living is involved in the tiredness. These types are almost too tired to sleep and the libido suffers as part of the general exhaustion. Use the 30c potency.

7) *Opium*
This is another remedy when fatigue and exhaustion dominates the sexual drive.

8) *Natrum mur.*
This remedy is essential at some time in the treatment whenever anxiety, fear and lack of confidence in the self is a dominant factor in the impotency. It must be used in the high 200c potency.

Frigidity
This is the female equivalent of masculine impotency. There is a tightness, rigidity and spasm of the vaginal muscles during the sexual act — often with vaginal anaesthesia — or there is felt to be a lack of the normal lubricants secreted during intercourse, which often is an added cause of tension and a barrier to response. In all cases there is a failure to achieve orgasm during the act, although this can be stimulated manually. There is a lack of normal vaginal sensitivity, due to apprehension concerning the male, and a paralyzing fear of being unable to adequately respond. Excitement in the partner serves to increase fear and tension rather than to act as a stimulus to pleasure and sensuality.

Such spasm and rigidity often reflects a tightness in the personality in certain areas, an inability to let go, to enjoy, to be a seductive woman and active sexual partner. With the help of education and the media, there has been a lessening of such constrictions in recent years, but in some the problem remains, and a manual orgasm is no solution for many women in an otherwise satisfactory relationship. For many women there is a sense of being much slower than the male to respond, often of not having enough time and of being under pressure, which also adds to tension and lessens excitement.

Sometimes such problems are a cause of depression and a sense of failure; or the problem may be denied and orgasm fabricated over the years, making for added difficulties since the problem is not shared, is less obvious than male potency difficulties, and can therefore be more easily ignored for longer periods. Yet it is only by discussion and patient tenderness that the difficulty can be cured, giving the possibility of a more open and confident, solid partnership with security, closeness and understanding. Once there is a more open attitude such intimate matters are more easily talked about and shared, leading quite naturally to more trust and confidence.

A major part of the problem is the common fear of losing control during orgasm and mounting excitement — the fear ultimately of being overwhelmed by feelings too intense to contain. This gives a sense of void during the sexual act, an overwhelming sensation which is both satisfying yet frustrating, taking the place of the more physical orgasm in a more controlled, yet remote, esoteric way. The male organ is both desired and feared and the intensity of this desire is both primitive and frightening, so that relaxation is difficult; giving way, enveloping and accepting becomes a thing of fear rather than of ecstasy and love.

Giving way is always the problem and often the woman has never really allowed herself to give way in any situation before because of her built-in controls. This applies equally to joy, laughter, tears or rage — both as a teenager and as a mature woman. She may have never properly rebelled as a teenager, never been fully herself, creating fear and lack of confidence in every situation. When there is not enough openness within the couple, resentments inevitably arise and underlying fears and problems tend to become more chronic, leading to deep feelings of depression, failure, non-fulfilment and often break-up of the relationship.

Recommended Remedies for Frigidity

1) *Pulsatilla*
This is indicated when there is a strong sexual interest, often to the point of being obsessional and intense; but however long the sexual act is prolonged these individuals are unable to achieve orgasm and often have to resort to manual satisfaction — which nearly always provokes feelings of failure and depression.

2) *Sepia*
There is total indifference to sexuality, often hostility to it, as all libidinal drive is undermined by a combination of dragging down back and uterine pains, constipation, exhaustion, irritability, depression and often a tendency to prolapse.

3) *Lachesis*
The sexual drive is often at a high level, but intercourse is painful and especially the left ovary is very tender, undermining organism.

4) *Natrum mur.*
This remedy is of special value when there are deep-seated fears of control and dependence and the inability to 'let go' in any situation. It is also of value in those cases of frigidity where the vaginal mucosa is excessively dry, so that the sexual act quickly becomes painful and

soreness develops which undermines any libidinal pleasures. For the deeper psychological problems, use the remedy in the 200c potency; for the problems of painful coitus due to mucosal dryness, use the 6c potency thrice daily.

Transvestitism

With few exceptions, this is almost entirely a masculine problem. The overwhelming desire is to dress in female clothes and is associated with a heightening of sexuality. In particular, female undergarments are of interest and sought after in order to produce the intense degree of excitement that in most cases leads to ejaculation. Dressing up is only a sexual perversion as long as it remains narcissistic and a masturbatory secret. When it is included within an adult relationship and made open it ceases to have any real power or signficance. The onset may be in the teens or earlier, as an aspect of adolescent sexuality and secret masturbation, excitement being heightened by possessing and then wearing clothing belonging to the masturbatory figure — usually a sister or mother.

A common feature of the dressing up is the looking or voyeuristic element. This usually involves looking at and admiring the self wearing the secret clothes, and is part of the narcissism and also competition and envy towards the other person involved in the phantasy. In general, the other person is felt to possess more attractive, lovable, desirable physical attributes than the male, and the aim is to possess such qualities for a temporary period in the mirror-image. Yet however exciting and magical the erotic formula may be, at the same time it is all too often seen through by the observing psyche, and felt to be a very poor second best to the original admired woman. Above all, it seems rather ridiculous and often sordid, which detracts from the pleasure of the moment and eventually weakens it entirely.

There are often strong infantile features, with childish phantasies and desires for comforts, searching to recreate earliest security and pleasures of warmth and closeness, particularly to the mother. The interest in rubber or leather stems from this very early period, and reflects the strength of such impulses to recapture the past, and to somewhat vainly relive them in phantasy. Because of this, there is a constant flight from the present, from adult burdens and responsibilities as they are imagined to be, because judgement of present contemporary reality is always weak. Mature sexual relationships are weak or totally absent, because so much of their energy is bound up with the past and their secret activities. In addition, guilt is inevitably associated with such activities because of the intense degree of narcissism involved.

Although sexuality may be present between the couple, in most cases it has broken down or has never been well established. The transvestite sexuality is always an intensely secret affair to the detriment of more mature sharing and intimacy in a couple. Often the undergarments of the wife are used in futile masturbatory bids to recapture infantile phantasy idealisms and a fleeting sense of belonging and completeness; at the same time shame and guilt are marked. The basic aim is to repeat a symbolic act in order to reassure — yet each act does the opposite and undermines any vestige of mature masculinity and self-respect that remains, in some ways making the act even more compulsive and futile.

When such activities occur in an engaged couple or within a marriage, there are invariably deep-seated problems. A truly sharing and therefore loving partnership is difficult to achieve, and the relationship is doomed to failure unless the problem can be discussed openly or treated professionally.

Dressing up may sometimes be a form of homosexual drag — an extension of a more severe break with masculinity and masculine identifications, and often a rejection of the father who is unconsciously punished for all his short-comings and failures. In such cases, any image of the son as the father would have wished him, is totally destroyed, and the identification is with the mother, although the wish is basically to punish the rejecting father and to shame him at the expense of fulfilment and growth. This is a double tragedy because it is really the father who was much admired and loved and who is now despised. Such feelings always come home to roost, creating sadness, confusion, futility and despair.

Recommended Remedies for Transvestitism

This is often a chronic intractable problem as a vestige of infantilism has taken over the whole of normal masculine development and identification because of earlier trauma or insecurity. The problem is one of immaturity and when it presents, the patient has often initially come with an entirely different complaint, especially depression or fears and insecurity.

1) *The Constitutional Remedy of the Individual*
I recommend that this be given initially in the 200c potency in order to stimulate psychological maturing and to increase confidence.

2) *Arnica*
There has nearly always been a psychological trauma in the earliest growth period — possibly indecent exposure or direct sexual molesting,

which itself has often been forgotten; the sexuality has been stimulated prematurely and excessively, creating a profound psychological shock though nearly always beyond recall. *Arnica* in the high 200c potency can help reverse this early shock and damage, and help to free stunted sexual growth and identification again.

3) *Sulphur*
When there is no initial response to treatment or if it seems slow I use *Sulphur* in the high potencies to unblock obscure areas of memory or fear where there is rigidity since this is why the remedies, though well indicated, fail to evoke sufficient response.

4) *A Nosode*
Medorrhinum or *Syphilinum* are of particular value, especially to follow the *Sulphur* remedy in a move to break down rigid attitudes and fears and to open up earlier psychological assumptions of an infantile type. Use once only in the 200c potency.

5) *Natrum mur.*
At some period in the treatment this great psychological remedy is always indicated, helping particularly with rigid assumptions, perceptions and attitudes which block maturity and growth. These individuals are nearly always 'loners', and the *Natrum mur.* helps facilitate more contact with others which is essential for psychological healing and development.

6) *Lycopodium*
This remedy has often given positive results, but only after the ground has been prepared as with the above remedies first.

Premature Ejaculation
Ejaculation either before or immediately after penetration is a frequent male problem. It always reflects masculine insecurity and anxiety which causes a heightened level of excitement so that the least act of intimacy or sexual approach may lead to a precipitate, uncontrolled ejaculation. This is often associated with depression, a sense of failure, an inevitable lack of confidence and a tendency to avoid contact with women who present any form of sexual challenge. The main feeling is of having no controls so that failure seems certain, with an added feeling of soiling and frustrating the woman so that the least approach will lead to rejection and loss. In such conditions, the male usually prefers to make no approach rather than risk failure and humiliation.

In general, women are idealized and seem unobtainable — placed on a pedestal, highly desired, yet powerful and threatening. Such feelings are invariably those of the small child towards the mother, which have remained unchanged in the adult. The sexual woman is seen only in primitive terms of demanding breasts or a vagina that wants immediate satisfaction, and will punish if not given in to. It is not surprising to note that such distorted imagery represents very much the demanding mouth greed of the small infant, insisting on immediate satisfaction, and indeed it is these fractions of infantile development that are now perceived in the woman and transform her into a powerful instrument of fear. Such strong unconscious elements psychologically create an impossible situation for the male because he at the same time feels inadequate, weak and small.

In all other areas, these men are often highly successful and achievers in the field of business or art. This success may be in part to compensate for feelings of sexual failure. They are often very generous — again to compensate for this area where they are unable to function; but the generosity is often with concrete, material things rather than with feelings and needs, which they tend to keep to themselves, often as an aspect of feeling vulnerable.

When in the company of other men, these individuals feel inferior, less successful and less manly, often competing in other fields such as business where they feel more secure. In nearly all areas they are highly individualistic, non-conformers and independent — needing to prove themselves superior in other ways by finding other, often creative solutions to a problem, but above all, always different and rarely part of a team. Often solitary, with a chip on their shoulder about some educational or early lack of experience, they tend to feel the need to be extremely provocative and challenging, never letting an argument go by in which they can prove a point and thereby themselves.

Beating records and targets in the work situation is common, and part of their drive is to be both different and better than the other man, leading to the enormous will to succeed. In business as in every situation, they are always seeking short-cuts so that they again create a pressure situation; they are rarely on time for anything — often too early for meetings — but above all short of time, so that whatever they do it has inevitably to be over too quickly — exactly as with their intimate situation. In almost every aspect of life they are short-fused, quick to flare up, or quick to show a tear, so that everything is eventually precipitate, hurried, and placed under pressure, especially when it involves any human contact with either men or women. Only when they are by themselves do these individuals take their time, and thus create equal frustration because nothing is ever quite ready or finished. Again a stressful situation arises, exactly like the sexual one; it may be the evening meal or a social engagement, when inevitably they must rush and leave late or do the impossible to arrive at all.

Remedies for Premature Ejaculation

1) *Lycopodium*
This is often the most valuable of all remedies, giving good results when the basic personality is one where everything — not just the sexuality — is rushed and precipitate. Because of a basic insecurity many of life's demands and challenges are left until the last moment, creating a pressure situation of anxiety and tension. This personality trait, combined with the general weakness in the inherent sexual drive creates the problem. It is important during treatment to help the patient see that this is not just a sexual problem but occurs in every facet of his being.

2) *Nux vomica*
The sexual drive is much more pronounced in this type than in the *Lycopodium* individual; it is often intense but because of the underlying psychological make-up, the very spasms of passion and the precipitateness inherent in the person, the pressures created can often bring about premature ejaculation. When they are able to relax and to be less intense there is usually no problem.

3) *Kalium phos.*
This remedy is associated with the quickness, the desire and the flashing intensity of the *Phosphorus* remedy, as well as the weakness and the lack of sexuality which characterizes the potassium element of the make-up. Such contradictions of desire often end in a non-event — the premature ejaculation — in spite of the positive intentions and interest.

Indecent Exposure
Public exposure of the male parts to the female is a very common form of sexual perversion and exhibitionism. It is always an expression of masculine inadequacy or depression, and is common in the 40-year age group, when the male is passing through a mid-life psychological period of adjustment and often crisis. Usually there has been a long-standing security problem with women, and such men have never been able to adequately form a deep, sharing heterosexual relationship. They tend to be either isolated, mother-dominated or, when married, the relationship

is a continuation of infancy, with the man in a childish, dependent and clinging position, rather than in the role of a supportive, sharing partner.

Sexuality is almost invariably weak or non-existent and the act of self-exposure is both a desperate attempt to make some contact with the woman, as well as an act of defiant rebuff and rebellion which was never allowed in the earlier years. The exposure is a frightening, compulsive act which evokes fear rather than reassurance, yet they are often unable to control the drive because of the sexual excitement in the situation and the fear and danger of being 'caught'.

Such 'flashers' present the erect organ to a strange woman, or sometimes to a child of either sex, who is not physically interfered with or attacked in the majority of cases. The exposure may be to a group of passing women in a car or coach, but the aim is always to show off, to frighten the victim, reassure himself and then usually to run away. Of course the act of exposure often does none of these things, and does nothing to bring about either confidence or growth. Usually, the act ends in compulsive masturbation with a sense of guilt and futility.

The act is always a very primitive and distorted one of a little boy wanting to show off to mother and to gain approval and attention — ultimately love. At the same time, the act also contains the expression of aggressive, ambivalent feelings, and this is why guilt and shame is prevalent. Such infantile displays in the adult give no hope of the sought-after love and attention ever developing, because it leads to increasingly isolation, depression and feelings of failure. Because the act tends to give little satisfaction, other than the degree of sexual excitement achieved, there is a compulsive need to repeat it, in order to try to overcome the sense of shame and inadequacy.

Recommended Remedies for Indecent Exposure
The problem may be recent in origin and of short duration, often following a clear-cut psychological trauma which the individual has not been able to contain and cope with. Stress or loss with denied grief are other common causes.

1) *The Constitutional Remedy of the Individual*
I recommend this initially in the 200c potency to strengthen underlying psychological aspects of the individual and to help bring to the surface and to cope with the true and deeper root causes.

2) *Platina*
This remedy is useful when there are overwhelming needs to display

and to show off in all areas including the sexual one. Pride is always marked, but the real and underlying problem is one of insecurity. Use in the 200c potency.

3) *Pulsatilla*

This remedy is indicated when there is a powerful need to be always on display which accounts for much of the shame and shyness. Voyeuristic needs are also strong — hence the blushing — and this is a significant element in the indecent display in that there is always a strong identification with the other person who is being made to look and is being subjected to the exposure. The underlying make-up and physiology must match that of the *pulsatilla* constitution in order for the remedy to be effective. Use in the 200c potency.

4) *Natrum mur.*

I use this remedy because it is associated with so many of the typical psychological elements of the indecent exposure make-up. There is fear of others and the avoidance of close contact; there is a preoccupation with sexuality that is often not shared or admitted to; *Natrum mur.* is linked with the furtiveness of the problem, and eye signs and involvement are marked because if the exposure is not seen, then it is not psychologically complete, is therefore a failure and has to be repeated.

17.

SCHIZOPHRENIA AND THE BREAK WITH REALITY

The schizophrenic illness is a common one and, without exception, serious whenever it occurs. Usually the cause is unknown, although often there is a family history of mental and emotional instability, eccentricity, or periods of confusion or break-down with or without hospitalization; such circumstances can often create increased pressure on the young developing personality. These hereditary factors, often in quite subtle ways, may be a cause of increased rigidity and intolerance by the family with inappropriate strictness or lack of caring at some of the most critical stages of upbringing and development.

In some cases there has been a prolonged trauma to both body and mind by the use of certain drugs, purchased either with or without prescription. The appetite suppressants have been one of the major culprits in recent years, causing instability and psychosis in some cases, in addition to the emotional displacement and underlying disturbance which was expressed in the compulsive addiction and drive to deal with all frustration and stress by eating. Over a prolonged period, with repeat prescriptions sometimes given over a period of years, there can be damage to the judgemental processes of the mind and the ability to differentiate reality from phantasy.

Another cause of the schizophrenic type of break-down is sometimes an acute physical trauma, as from an industrial accident with loss of a limb. In a rigid personality the shock may be so great as to be overwhelming, and an acute delusional psychosis can suddenly occur without warning and with no previous history of mental break-down. Also the sudden loss of a job, due to redundancy or liquidation, the break-down of a marriage, with a difficult and prolonged divorce, can in a phobic or obsessional type of personality tip the balance from relatively simple claustrophobic fears into an acutely delusional state with complete loss of all reason and insight. There are some families who live under a great deal of emotional disturbance and tension with considerable dissension, anger and frustration which is never permitted to come out openly and be dealt with in a healthy way.

In such families, often with a history of mental disturbance which may have occurred in a previous generation, a particularly vulnerable and often quiet and withdrawn member seems to be at the centre of all the underlying tensions and indeed to contain much of it, thereby preventing a total split within the family, but at the cost of his own health and sometimes sanity. A situation of 'double-bind' is created, where the individual in question can neither express his feelings openly without provoking a dangerous family crisis and the threat of fragmentation, nor can he leave and save himself, because his departure would apparently stimulate an even worse crisis. Such fears and certainties of the impossibility of change are stimulated by the individual's own phantasies and by many subtle, unconscious and often more definite threats by the family as to what might 'happen' if he were to leave. In such a situation, after holding the family together over many months or years, appearing 'normal' because so much is kept hidden or denied, suddenly there is a complete break-down and the rather vague, withdrawn state becomes one of delusional belief and unreality.

In a non-psychotic emotional situation, however healthy the family or the individual, there are nevertheless remnants of earlier traumas and scars of old hurts. Although these do not dominate the personality or the relationships formed within the family or outside it, these traces must be resolved and dealt with. The 'normal' way of dealing with such neurotic fragments from the past is by 'working through' them in a social situation. Problems of jealousy, sibling rivalry, hurt and loss are recreated within a working situation or everyday relationship and the figures from the past with many of the old unresolved feelings come to the surface — illogically perhaps — but in a new yet similar adult situation where they can be modified and understood more easily by the more mature adult mind. The common office tensions, rivalries, hates and dislikes as well as the support and friendships made in most cases are an important aspect of this 'working through' process as well as contributing to some of the inevitable tensions and discussions or difficulties that occur; often this process is the reason for an excessive amount of time to be taken over deciding a seemingly simple problem.

I call this non-psychotic resolution of tense emotional areas the 'social' or 'normal' *Simillimum* principle because the individual creates in their social environment a traumatic situation similar to that of his infancy — in most cases — and can then more easily come to terms with it. In this way, areas of the personality where growth has been blocked by old resentments and hurts can be released quite naturally and the natural process of maturity can continue.

There is also a 'neurotic' *Simillimum* process, whereby the same type of underlying emotional areas of hurt, resentment, rivalry or loss are re-experienced in adult life by creating similar figures and personalities at work or in any other situation. But here there is far too much intensity of feeling to allow any real growth or coming-to-terms to occur. All the ingredients of the earlier situation are re-enacted with great drama and feeling causing alienation, unpopularity and a further repeat of the initial hurt. Because of the neurotic reaction, any working through is slow as compared with the more benign 'social' *Simillimum* process.

The psychotic cannot work through or express his underlying problems, either by the social or the neurotic *Simillimum* principle, because of the severity of his illness and the fragmented and often threatening world of the schizophrenic.

Within the schizophrenic mind, everything is fragmented and largely unrelated to any logical order. The fragments of self, mind and phantasy are always placed outside the self and, by a process of psychological projection, experienced as alien to the person and not part of it. Thus a bewildering, kaleidoscopic world of fact, phantasy, delusion, hallucination and suspicion is created, with the frequent impression of ideas of reference where others are felt to be looking at them or talking about them, passing comments or sending messages over the radio or television. Any form of integrative 'knitting together' of earlier trauma in a harmonious way cannot occur because the whole energy and drive of the schizophrenic is towards the outside, towards splitting away, denial, fragmentation and disharmony. Inevitably, this leads to chaos of both self image and those of others.

The core of schizophrenia is always damage to the ego or self feeling — the ability to differentiate self from environment, as the psychotic process seems to invade and to break down the boundary or sense of where the body and mind begins and ends. The patient experiences both inner and exterior sensations as a continuum and sees no barrier between them so that confusion is marked.

The psychotic cannot effect a normal *Simillimum* cure in a social situation because he denies his very existence and identity as an individual. The psychotic process pulverizes both his experience of the outer world and its personalities and relationships, as well as that of the inner world with all its elements of mind, thought and feelings, into a confused mixture of disorganized fragments. It is these fragments that become the world, the experience and the perceptions of the schizophrenic.

The essential nature of the illness is this projection of self, its fragments and images of self into outside situations, whilst creating a break with reality and a world of delusion and unreality. Such feelings create a sense of bewilderment, depression, of being dead and empty inside, emotionally flat to the outsider, unable to respond or to relate in any appropriate or straightforward way which has any meaning or sense. The difference between this and the depressive state is that whatever the phantasies of death or destruction, there is no severe degree of psychotic projection and therefore no break with reality.

This basic splitting off and projection of fragments of the self is the cause of all the schizophrenic 'madness', inappropriate hallucinations and feeling of being on a different wave-length. The external world of the psychotic is not one of sibling rivalry, parental frustration or jealousy, but one of fragments often felt to be living inside others, felt to contain aspects of his most personal and private thoughts and feelings. Much of this is responsible for the delusional belief that others can read his thoughts and mind or also that he can omnipotently know what others are saying and thinking. Only when these dispersed fragments of the self are acknowledged as part of the self and gathered back within the psychic envelope, is a cure possible, so that the boundaries of the self may be strengthened and made intact again.

One of the problems of the psychotic is that anyone in contact with this type of personality quickly becomes part of his delusional world and this includes the homoeopathic physician and any prescribed remedies, which can easily become objects of suspicion and mistrust. There is nearly always the slow and difficult problem of gaining the patient's confidence and overcoming the barrier of hostility. There must be co-operation from the more healthy and amenable parts of the person in order for the treatment to have a chance of acting, as otherwise the remedies are hidden or thrown away; it maybe necessary to wait until an acute crisis has passed before beginning a treatment.

All of us contain opposing tendencies, being both self-destructive as well as creative in our feelings, thinking, urges and expressions of need. The main features of the illness are withdrawal, unreality and delusional conviction, as the self-destructive urges overwhelm both understanding and creative thought which is essentially healthy and reparative, more balanced and less distorted.

The acute psychotic illness is a disturbing one for patient and family alike. If it occurs in the early years, the previous personality has usually been somewhat withdrawn, shy and quiet. There is a great intensity about everything, coupled with a make-up which is at best highly individualistic, and often has a bizarre quality to it; the personality is somewhat eccentric and has a tendency to withdrawal from much personal contact. As the illness develops, there is usually a further withdrawl into the self so that symptoms and ideas become increasingly unreal and unstable.

There is a return to the almost total 'magical' thinking or dreaming of the obsessional illness. In this case it is more widespread and accompanied by hallucination. The disease process creates a mixture of primitive magical and mythological thinking — very much the basic symbols and language of the dream and or art, particularly that of surrealism and Blake, Dali and Jung.

In the acute phase, particularly when the patient is over-active to an extreme degree, the family may provide an important clue to the choice of remedy when the patient is too disturbed to be co-operative for reasons of acute mistrust and suspicion. Because the homoeopathic remedy acts at both a physical as well as an emotional level, this can foster a relationship between physician and the schizophrenic patient. The well-prescribed remedy helps the patient sufficiently in many cases to allow the physician to relate more easily with his more healthy personality areas which have not been fragmented. Even when these areas seem initially to be only remnants of a person, they can be strengthened and stimulated to grow into more positive areas of self.

Before discussing the more definite homoeopathic prescribing, I would like to look more closely at three examples of hallucinatory material from a 23-year-old schizophrenic girl, with a four-year history of agoraphobia, a fear of all women but especially of her mother, and a symptom of having heard voices for six months. She also had a certainty that others were talking about her in a critical way. During her visits, she was largely silent, smiling and giggling inappropriately, looking at the ceiling. Eventually on the fourth meeting and after the constitutional remedy had been prescribed, she volunteered the following details of her hallucinations: 'Let's get together! The doctors stink.', and finally 'Eat, don't talk, eat.'

My comments about 'Let's get together' were that they did not only relate to her getting together with me in a working relationship where the homoeopathic treatments could help her, but also to her getting together as a person and her wish for that to happen, so that the healthy part of her could heal all the splits and distortions which caused so much muddle and confusion. I said also that because of the illness, she was experiencing aspects and parts of herself talking to her from outside, and that although she found it secretly amusing, it must also distress her and frighten her at times. It was these voices — parts of her own functioning and psychology which had got pushed away and outside her which she wanted back inside to make her feel more whole again. Most of my emphasis here was placed on the healthy integrative impulses coming from her healthy personality remnant, relating and encouraging it, rather than emphasizing her contact with me — although this was not less important.

The second piece of hallucinatory material — namely 'The doctors stink' — was put to her as a reflection of her ill self, felt to be bad, rotten, putrid and unloving because it was unused and unexpressed, as if shut away. This made her feel unattractive and undesirable to others. By making me — the 'doctors' — stink, she was attempting to put this aspect of herself outside herself and into me as one of the doctors, but at the same time was creating more confusion and less 'getting together'.

The third piece of hallucination — 'Eat, don't talk, eat' was linked to her making herself a receptacle for food, a sort of dustbin lacking identity, rather than acknowledging herself as a person with feelings and ideas. The patient was very obese with a greasy, unhealthy skin and this worried her. She would like to have been slim like her younger sister — a full-time student. Talking and words were ways of making contact and closeness, but because she distrusted people and was unsure of them and their motives, she preferred to eat, thereby losing the contacts with others which could help her.

If we now look more closely at adolescent schizophrenia, it is clear that not only are there mental changes, but also physical ones. The skin is often damp from a generalized perspiration and the extremities are frequently icy cold. There is often a greasy quality to the skin, particularly that of the forehead, chin, shoulders and back which may provoke a severe acne and tendency to blackheads. Dandruff is common and a cause of anxiety in an adolescent gaining confidence in their appearance. Obesity is a frequent problem due to a liking for greasy, starchy, fattening goods. For such temperaments *Calcarea carb.* is often indicated as their constitutional treatment and a basis for the homoeopathic approach to the psychotic problem.

The bulky, overweight adolescent, greasy-skinned, and with a damp, sweaty skin, especially over the forehead, and often with cold hands and feet generally requires *Calcarea* at some point in his treatment, particularly if there is a combination of fidgety restlessness and associated body weakness and pallor. They are usually very thirsty individuals and often drink a sweet, milky tea throughout the day, as well as usually hugging the fire. *Calcarea sulph.* may be indicated when the patient is warmer, is very untidy and has an early morning aggravation of the mental symptoms. Often they express the paleness and the bulky build of *Calcarea* together with the sweaty heat and love of fats of the *Sulphur* remedies.

There is another form of adolescent schizophrenia which is commonly seen in the consulting room. These are nearly always slim and anorexic girls, with a grossly distorted body image, obsessed by food and diet, the extremities cold, blue or damp from sweating, with constant problems of weakness and exhaustion. When there is an added problem of chronic infection anywhere in the body, with a tendency to boils or pus formation, then *Silicea* may relieve both the physical and the mental problems.

In the psychotic patient, however disturbed, there is always a healthy residual part of the person which is able at times to relate to others at a reality level and is not lost to the schizophrenic process. No matter how deluded, there are periods when he is sensible and able to make contact in a meaningful way with his environment. Business acumen and skill is not necessarily undermined until the disease is severe and judgement becomes distorted and, until then, the schizophrenic may function without any severe problems. During a period of reality, he exists as an entity, makes contact with others and can recognize others as separate beings from himself, individuals in their own right. Such sense of existence and boundaries may be weak but it is not fragmented, as in the acute schizophrenic process.

It is this healthy part, healthy residue, that is the seed of recovery for the schizophrenic, providing that the disease process is not too destructive. In treating the psychotic, it is important to acknowledge and to strengthen this positive integrating part of the self without denying the sick self. The homoeopathic remedy in highest potency acts directly upon it to strengthen and to widen it. Between myself and the unfragmented ego, I attempt to build a bridge of trust, openness and discussion, in order that both the patient and I can discuss and relate anything either he or I considers relevant. I always find it useful to discuss dreams as well as hallucinatory material in the consultations, in an attempt to understand the mental state together and also to share it more with the unaffected ego. Much of this is of direct concern and interest to the patient, and often creates anxiety and at times confusion.

Whatever is related is accepted and discussed in terms of the fragmentation process and the remedy prescription. At the same time, this lays emphasis on the healthy move towards integration and cure, even though this seems in no way possible or obvious in a period of acute flare up. Often the patient's dreams give the clue to how the integrated side of the patient is developing and how he is coping with the onslaught of the fragmentation process. At all times, the physical symptoms and general health must be taken into consideration as a guideline and confirmatory factor for the correct remedy.

Some authorities, in particular R. D. Laing, have described the 'explorative voyage' aspect of the schizophrenic process; this is a voyage into knowing and is an essential and inevitable part of the disturbed individual's growth and unity as a person, faced with a crisis in his life that cannot be resolved other than by almost complete break-down. Only when the person has reduced himself to the very basis and foundations of his identity can he be 'reconstructed' as a more healthy and creative, less rigid and blocked personality, with a greater depth of understanding of himself and others.

The essential nature of the schizophrenic process can only be true when the previous personality, family circumstances and relationships were so rigidly confined and strict, that life was unbearable and that a turbulent psychotic breakdown was the only way out of an unlivable reality. In such a desperate situation, there is a total fragmentation into the component parts of the person, and these can be widely dispersed before being gathered again in a stronger and more ordered form as the person emerges with more potential and greater freedom for creativity — ultimately for giving, loving and developing.

The Paranoid Personality

There is an attitude of mind, seen from adolescence onwards in certain personalities, which is a precursor of a possible break-down, although at the time there is no break with reality. With the paranoid personality everything is seen in terms of possible criticism or hostility. Often it only comes to the surface after a hurt or situation of rejection, although often such hurts and rejections are either distorted or created by the individual to confirm that people are against him and not to be trusted. The main problem is a paranoid attitude, with a sudden and very intense feeling of being attacked, or devalued in some way. Such reactions are very frequent and never far from the surface, intruding into every relationship to some degree. Usually there is an aggressive, cutting response to such supposed criticisms; rejection is severe, and such aggression is justified by the demeaning attitudes of others.

In general, a misunderstanding leads on quickly to a rapid spiral of destructive behaviour, withdrawal and a most negative and unwarranted outburst. These personalities often feel themselves to be failures and although they desire closeness, there is an inability to see misunderstandings and temporary difficulties in any way other than in the most extreme and hostile terms. Constantly they feel criticized and rejected and despair of ever finding anyone capable of caring. Often there have been previous break-downs, periods of severe depression or suicidal attempts and delusional conviction is never far from the surface.

The Paranoid Position

Usually this is a very severe mental illness of the 40-year age group. There is a powerful delusional process, either coming on slowly over the years or sometimes acutely after a sudden and devastating accident or traumatic shock — for instance, after a road accident, concussion and head injury, or loss of limb. But in most cases the cause is not known and the onset is slow and gradual, often in a seemingly normal personality, with a tendency to the paranoid personality make-up

In the paranoid illness there is a marked increase in rigid thinking and conceptions of others and their motivations. There is also isolation and certitude of beliefs. Suspicions and notions of being hard done by or singled out for unfair treatment are common as is a sense of being made an example of, leading to frequent outbursts of passionate anger. The certitude of having been singled out and specially selected for persecution and punishment is characteristic and the illness itself and its treatment is felt to be part of a devilish plot and attack which is being wrongly dealt them. Quite frequently, the paranoid individual is convinced as to who is behind the plots to discredit him or to have him certified insane in order to get rid of him. Such people often include the secret service, MI5, the CIA, or the KGB. These delusions also have their dangerous side, and in some cases the illness may lead either to suicide or at other times to dangerous and sometimes fatal attacks on the imagined persecutors, especially when the delusion is confined to just one contemporary person. The family, the doctors, in fact anyone in the immediate environment is treated with suspicion and mistrust, as possible members of the plot. But beneath the surface, such powerful delusions are often based on envy of success and feelings of inadequacy and depressing failure; the feelings compensated for by the individual in making himself the object of so much persecutory attention, indirectly emphasizing his importance, rather than sense of failure and despair.

It is rare for such feelings to be admitted to, however, or for any closeness or intimacy to be allowed. There may be a few trusted people, but ultimately even the appearance of friendliness is suspect, and is seen as a possible ruse to get more information out of them. Often these personalities suddenly 'turn the tables' and show that they are 'not fools' and that they really know who the others are working for and who is their master. Quite often the somewhat grandiose associations, the name-dropping, their sphere of knowledge and influence have a reality base to a certain degree, because not uncommonly they have been highly successful and often influential in the past before the break-down. But this is not always true either and for others the whole delusional plot has no foundations in experience or previous contacts.

Although it is generally kept secret by the individuals concerned, they feel themselves to be at the centre of a unique and fantastic plot, the victims of an omnipotent power which all too clearly represents their own self-destructiveness, turned against them. There is a common tendency to withdraw and to become a loner as fewer people are trusted, so that he meditates upon his own fate and on those who are plotting against him. There may be counter-plots of revenge or a tendency to complain and to suffer unceasingly from the injustice of it all. They feel that they can have no real rest with safety, only interference by hallucinations and delusional thoughts. At times the delusions become grandiose and unreal in the extreme, feeling that they are Messiahs; that they expiate the sins of the worlds, or are being crucified by their problems and persecutors; that they are on their own against the world, and its attempts to destroy them.

The Action of Homoeopathy in Schizophrenia

Homoeopathy is always helpful in schizophrenia; in certain cases it is curative. Most cases treated have shown a lessening of over-activity and frequently the sleep disturbances have improved markedly. Often the main problem is the initial one of persuading the patient to accept both doctor and treatment. When this can be overcome, depending upon the severity and length of the illness, the outlook is a positive one. It is not uncommon to see a lessening of hallucinations as the patient begins to take an interest in his appearance again, frequently neglected in the acute phase of the illness.

The patient is often worried about his general health and appearance, and particularly in the case of young or adolescent patients, who are concerned with their hair, weight and general energy. With the homoeopathic prescription, it is common to see an improvement in the health of the skin and hair at an early stage with a lessening of acne or infection. Constipation is another area of anxiety and preoccupation, and this also usually improves at an early stage. As the patient makes some progress in terms of general health and vitality, this reassures him about the doctor and his treatment, lessens the underlying sense of defeat and hopelessness, and allows more time for the deep-acting mental remedies to work.

The eminent homoeopath Paschero, in a 1975 paper on mental symptoms in homoeopathy states that the homoeopathic *Simillimum* remedy 'stimulates the natural forces of the fundamental man and makes possible a rectification of his vital senses.' The importance of empathy and the doctor-patient understanding and relationship is emphasized.

He also states that the correct constitutional remedy may be the solution to many of the biological or deep-seated constitutional mental problems, and these were demanded so urgently by Freud for many of his more difficult and disturbed cases. Such cases with fundamental biological problems are often the schizophrenic ones, where the constitutional remedy in high potency can begin to re-establish the personality and the way back to integration and cure.

Recommended Remedies for Schizophrenia
In all cases, it is of primary importance to choose a remedy which best fits the presenting and dominant mental symptoms at the time of prescription and which also fits the major physical charateristics, symptoms and modalities. The individual constitutional remedy in at least the 200c potency is of primal importance at an early stage in the treatment.

Considering the basic remedies which may be of value in the schizophrenic condition, it is important to remember the three remedies recommended by Nash in the treatment of over-excitable manic psychosis. These are *Belladonna, Stramonium* and *Hyoscyamus*.

1) *Belladonna*
This is the extract from the deadly nightshade plant at the time of flowering in summer, and is of value when there is a pseudo-psychosis secondary to infection, with delirium or alcoholism. There is a remittent fever and the typical redness of the skin, particularly the face, together with complaints of heat and dryness. Burning pains and a rapid pounding pulse are common. This remedy is of most value when there is violent, uncontrollable manic excitement, great restlessness, delusional beliefs leading to over-activity, violence and halluncinations. When both the physical symptoms are present with the uncontrollable excitement, there is a positive and calming response.

2) *Stramonium*
This remedy is made from the entire plant of the Thorn Apple and treats many of the most severe and problematic symptoms of schizophrenia. It is of value when there are bouts of excitability, extreme restlessness and the most agitated delusional activity. Compared with the symptoms associated with *Belladonna*, the fever is continual rather than intermittent, there is less redness and the patient is talkative and over-active to an extreme degree.

3) *Hyoscyamus*

This is the extract of the plant Henbane. It is not usually linked with fever and is characterized by passive delirium with halluncinations, suspicion, and many obsessional features, the patient lying picking at the bed-clothes, out of touch with reality.

4) *Tarantula hisp.*

This remedy is the extract of the entire insect, found along the Mediterranean coast. It is used for the most destructive of all the schizophrenic types when there is soiling, tearing of bed-clothes or clothes, and attempts at self-destruction, often highly dangerous. Mood changes are always excessive and rapid with swings from hypermania to the depths of despair. In all cases where the remedy is indicated, there is always marked agitation.

5) *Thuja occidentalis*

This is known as the tree of life and is prepared from the young leaves picked at the end of June. It is a well tried remedy for many bizarre and hypochondriacal symptoms. Depression is predominant and there is a tendency to agitation, anxiety and often irritability with fixed delusional ideas. These delusions are often odd and peculiar to the extreme — for instance, there may be a feeling that the body is brittle, transparent, made of glass and will shatter at the least shock. At times these patients feel that they have a live animal in their bowels, or there is pain in one localized and particular spot like 'nails being driven through the head'. Often they feel influenced by a superior power. The association of fig warts or condylomata, especially in the anal area, confirms the remedy and diagnosis.

6) *Anacardium orientale*

This is made from the fruit of the tree. There are many disturbed features associated with this remedy: hallucinations, a sense of split personality, feeling divided by contradictory impulses or controlled and commanded by an external force. There are many strange and obsessional features too and loss of memory is common. The patient laughs inappropriately at voices and hallucinations. There are two odd diagnostic symptoms: a) a feeling of having a plug in the inner parts — head, chest, navel or anus; b) a sense of there being a hoop around the body and encircling it.

7) *Lachesis*

This remedy is indicated for suspicion and paranoia, combined with mild over-activity. There is a total inability to tolerate pressure about the neck or chest and, characteristically, the patient sleeps into an aggravation of the mental state, waking from sleep in a more severe and agitated frame of mind. Nearly all symptoms of hallucination and over-activity are worse in the morning. Usually there is a tendency to depression and melancholia, yet the individual is talkative at the same time. When there is pain and discomfort, it is nearly always left-sided.

Psora is the name given to the inherited streak or tendency to certain patterns of illness, called a miasm, or 'ghost of illness', which Hahnemann described in his writings on chronic illness and its treatment. This disease complex called psora has many bizarre, chronic refractory problems and symptoms, but especially prevalent are mental disease and delusions of all kinds. In a difficult, refractory, non-responsive case, this diagnosis must not be forgotten. Of all the anti-psora remedies, probably *Sulphur* and *Psorinum* are the most valuable. *Causticum* is also of value, but especially the first two remedies are often needed when well indicated remedies fail to elicite a healing response.

18.

TENSION STATES AND IRRITABILITY

One of the commonest emotional problems seen in any surgery is the state of tension, often inseparable from an anxiety state. It is, however, always a physical state with an underlying emotional cause. Commonly there is an awareness of an emotional block, an underlying problem that cannot be dealt with or easily discussed for reasons of the personalities concerned, or because of the limitations of the communication permitted in the relationship. A real or imagined barrier is present, which cannot be overcome and which is the cause of the tension and heightened feelings, provoking an imbalance in normal muscular relaxation and tone with a mixture of emotional and physiological changes; these form the typical picture of the tension state. Everything is held in that wants naturally to burst out — hence the tension, anxiety and discomfort. Because the smooth, unconsciously controlled muscles respond to the state of health and equilibrium of the emotions, they are the main target and receptors for imbalance and heightened tension, translating emotional blockages and frustrations into physical symptoms. These occur wherever the unconscious has a powerful sphere of physical influence and representation by way of smooth muscles — particularly affected are the stomach, colon, walls of blood vessels, chest and sometimes the joints of limbs or lower back region.

Restlessness, either physical or emotional is common, leading to the general symptom of physical exhaustion and fatigue. Because of the state of agitation, the need to move, change position, to find a comfort that seems to exist nowhere, insomnia is always a problem and adds to the general anxiety and state of exhaustion. Tension does not cease during the night, and often the person wakes to find himself grinding his teeth, and with a fixed jaw and body. Nightmares are a frequent occurrence, often with a feeling of being trapped or attacked, with no possibility of escape, to such a degree at times that sleep itself is feared, in spite of the fatigue. In the sensitive young child, sleep-walking may occur, the child sometimes impossible to wake.

Backache is common, usually in the low lumbar region, often intractible, sometimes chronic, and made worse by a variety of treatments that do not sufficiently acknowledge the underlying emotional causes and allow them to emerge. This low back pain also interferes with sleep, as does worry about indigestion and sometimes constipation; the whole of the intestinal system becomes blocked and sluggish like the mental state. In others the bowels react more violently and there are bouts of diarrhoea, which may develop into the more severe colitis when the walls of the intestine ulcerate and blood is present in the stools, with the risk of infection or perforation occurring in a severe state. In such cases the very physical response seems to become a thing in its own right, cut off from the original tension state, and almost replacing it in significance. The other problem that is common is asthma in the sensitive adult or child. Here again the symptoms may develop a life and energy of their own however the underlying tensions evolve and are treated.

A tension state may become intolerable as tension and emotion builds up which cannot be adequately expressed. There may be a complete nervous break-down and, instead of a psychosomatic state developing as outlined above, there is a sudden catharsis of hysterical screaming, violent behaviour and the risk of a suicidal gesture as an expression of the mixed feelings of rage and tension.

Not uncommonly the tension state is complicated further by its treatment. When the tension is severe, almost invariably the allopathic drug treatment is unsatisfactory, provoking problems of dependence, fatigue, heaviness of waking and lethargy. Tension may be even further heightened by the inevitable tranquillizers, which all too often pose an added problem for the patient by provoking similar side-effects of tension and anxiety to those they aim to relieve.

Because of the degree of agitation, the feelings of exhaustion and the inability to concentrate, the patient usually needs a period away from work. As so much of the energy is taken up with anxiety about his symptoms, problems and how to resolve them, a self-centred preoccupation may develop, becoming hypochondriacal if not resolved. The problem with a chronic tension state is always that if it is not resolved within a period of several weeks by the release and resolution of the underlying emotional state, the physical symptoms become much more set in a pattern, and may be impossible to resolve.

A certain degree of tension and awareness is normal in everyone, and is part of healthy anticipation and attentiveness. Adrenalin is released to stimulate body tone in anticipation of a challenge or possible action.

Lack of tone and tension leads to an unhappy state of flabbiness, a sluggish ungainly posture and lack of energy as opposed to more compact flowing movements. This lack of tone is associated with accident-proneness, clumsiness and often hormonal imbalance, and is an indication for such homoeopathic remedies of the carbonate family as *Calcarea* or *Kalium carb.* The absence of tone is no more healthy than an excess of muscular tone, as is characteristic of the typical tension state. Anger is perfectly normal for all people yet it is a reaction which is often suppressed and denied because it is feared; in this way natural assertiveness is often the victim of our present upbringing, although essential to health. For the majority, it is the total absence of aggression which is the major problem provoking the build-up of severe tension states.

The internalization and denial of frustration does not stop the constant release of adrenalin, causing a heightening of body tone, an outpouring of blood sugar, with no possible outlet for the energy. Inevitably, this leads to mental and physical ill health, such dangerous conditions as diabetes or peptic ulcer, and general malaise and irritability as all outlets are denied. This excess of body tension is always produced by unresolved feelings of conflict, either conscious or unconscious. The net result is invariably heightened feelings of apprehension and a tightening of tension in any part of the body; particularly the chest, abdomen and back are prone to the development of pain.

Recommended Remedies for Tension States

1) *The Constitutional Remedy*
I give this initially, whenever possible, to free any underlying rigidity so that subsequent remedies have more available energy or charge to allow them to act. The results are usually obvious to the patient which naturally increases a state of relaxation, confidence and an increased confidentiality and trust which allows deeper causes to emerge and to be looked at.

2) *Natrum mur.*
I usually give this remedy in high potency early in the treatment and inevitably it has to be repeated — sometimes several times as progress is made. It has the capacity to reduce withdrawal and isolation, to reduce fear of others (unless based on a delusional assumption — when other remedies are indicated) and to facilitate contact with others, including the physician. In this way it makes for growth and a lessening of fear

and tension. The 200c potency is essential.

3) *Argentum nit.*
Indicated when there are overriding problems of obsessional fear or phobia which contribute to the tension state and prolong it through often long-standing phantasy ideas and distortions of the world and others, creating an overwhelming threat to normal functioning and severe tension.

4) *Gelsemium*
There is a combination of weakness and fear, especially of anything that is about to happen. This creates unbearable and paralyzing tension, exhaustion and often attacks of nervous diarrhoea.

5) *Arsenicum*
A remedy for an acute state of tension, to such a degree that the whole body becomes restless and overactive particularly in the early hours when sleep may be disturbed at about 1.00 a.m.

6) *Tuberculinum*
There is a chronic tension, and the person only finds relief from movement — doing something, or often from travelling. The symptoms are often worse in the evening. Give once only in the 200c potency.

7) *Carbo veg.*
Use for chronic tension states with extreme tremor and anxiety.

Anger and Irritability
Irritability and anger are not necessarily unhealthy unless excessive or uncontrollable. Such feelings occur at some time from birth onwards since frustration and pain are inevitably a part of life and at the same time inseparable from some degree of anger. The young child has many problems to cope with which are often painful and unpleasant, and not easy to understand. These include teething and weaning, the arrival of another 'rival' baby, all of which can lead to infantile rage as attention and comfort are felt to be interfered with, leading to a sense of deprivation. In later years, anger and irritability accompany different, more adult painful conditions, which limit the sense of well-being as with the common diseases of society, especially chronic catarrh seen from infancy onwards, headache, also present at all ages, and the omnipresent lumbago and backache, which affects nearly every adult male, whatever the occupation. In spite of the plethora of antibiotics,

sprays and antihistamines available, many children are chronically undermined by the most acute and painful recurrent ear infections, or those involving the throat and tonsils, often made worse by repetitive treatments; they cause considerable misery and spasms of pain and rage are both common.

Painful physical problems act as triggers to set off patterns of response of the underlying personality. Such patterns are of rigid construction, so that there is a 'short fuse', poor control, little resilience and set attitudes. Basic confidence is weak, the ego too easily shaken and uncertain. In order to cover up such uncertainties, there is a tendency to be over-assertive, often with fervour and an intense dislike at being disagreed with. These attitudes are particularly common for the person of *Nux vomica* make-up. In addition, there is often an underlying depression, with feelings of frustration, futility and uncontrolled outbursts towards the self as well as others. When such outbursts occur in middle age, and are out of keeping with previous attitudes and behaviour, then a general check-up is essential to exclude organic disease, which in some cases presents at an early stage by personality changes.

Because of the general state of tension and irritability, everything about the person, including his relationships with others, is generally too quick and too intense, with little real awareness, satisfaction and pleasure as the true energy of the body is repressed and expressed indirectly. In a sense everything is over before it is started. Sexual satisfaction is also minimal, primarily because of the lack of giving and sensitivity and feelings of involvement or caring.

Food is never really savoured and enjoyed, but rather devoured and eaten far too rapidly — hence the frequent complaints of heartburn pain and indigestion. Food is often not even tasted or recalled, there is no stimulation of the taste buds and it is swallowed and gulped and forced down without saliva, hence the acidity occurring shortly afterwards. The bowels are constipated because the food is not properly digested, because the diet is unbalanced and because of the underlying stress and tension.

Recommended Remedies for Anger and Irritability

It is important to remember that an angry reaction is often one of depression or of being unsure how to cope in any other way with a situation that seems to present a threat. It is a very surface reaction and is not only to 'let off steam', but equally to control and manipulate others. Particularly morning irritability may cover morning 'blues' Unless the underlying problems are resolved, the anger is likely to persist. In many cases, whoever is on the receiving end, it is nearly always directed at the self.

1) *Nux vomica*
Spasms of anger and irritability are common, usually short-lasting, with poor self-control and high standards. Indigestion and backache are often physical manifestations of the underlying tension.

2) *Chamomilla*
A well-known infantile remedy, but also indicated in adult anger. There is marked irritability, with a demanding need for attention and to be held and comforted. As soon as the individual is left for a moment the anger and demands start up again.

3) *Cina*
This remedy is indicated when the individual is irritable to the extent of wanting to hit or lash out at those around him. In general, he is restless and wants to be left alone — any attention or attempts to comfort makes him more irritable.

4) *Staphisagria*
This is recommended for an angry resentful personality with feelings of sometimes uncontrollable yet suppressed anger and indignation — hurt pride, wanting to burst out and to exact revenge, yet controlled, causing many physical problems.

5) *Colocynthis*
There is a combination of rage, indignation and hurt pride, causing a severe state of colic and restlessness.

6) *Sepia*
There is a mixture of anger and painful exhaustion at the end of the day. Everything drags this individual down— his job, chores, family, and he can be bothered with none of it. Indifferent, worn-out and depressed, the only thing that can possibly lift their irritability is dancing.

LIST OF
RECOMMENDED REMEDIES

Aconitum
Anacardium orientale
Agaricus
Argentum nit.
Arnica
Arsenicum alb.
Asafoetida
Aurum met.

Baptisia
Baryta carb.
Belladonna
Borax
Bryonia

Cactus
Cadmium phosp.
Calcarea
Cannabis indica.
Capsicum
Causticum
Chamomilla
China
Cicuta
Cimicifuja racemosa
Cina
Coffea
Colocynthis
Cuprum met.

Cyclamen

Drosera

Gelsemium
Graphites

Helleborus
Hyoscyamus

Ignatia
Iodum

Kali. carb.

Lac deflor.
Lachesis
Lilium tig.
Lycopodium

Mag. carb.
Medorrhinum
Medusa
Moschus

Naja
Natrum mur.
Natrum sulph.
Nitric acid

Nux moschata
Nux vomica

Opium

Passiflora
Phosphoric acid
Phosphorus
Plumbum
Pulsatilla

Rhus tox.

Sepia
Silicea
Staphisagria
Stramonium
Sulphur

Tarantula hisp.
Thuja
Thyroidinum
Tuberculinum

Valerian
Veratrum alb.

Zincum met.

INDEX

Other titles from Healing Arts Press
for further reading on homeopathy…

HOMEOPATHIC MEDICINE
A Doctor's Guide to Remedies for Common Ailments
Trevor Smith, M.D.
ISBN 0-89281-293-1
$9.95 paperback

This useful guide demonstrates that homeopathic care can encompass hundreds of ailments and first-aid needs, including care and treatment of childhood illness, difficulties of adolescence, acute illnesses of adults and adult couples, challenges of middle age, and the special needs of the elderly. A practicing physician, homeopath, and psychiatrist, Dr. Smith is sensitive to the delicate psychological problems that occur in each age group, and he places equal emphasis on the physical and mental aspects of health, stressing the importance of an open-minded approach and attitude toward illness. This detailed, self-help guide is an indispensable reference for home health care.

"…offers some of the most useful self-care information around. Looking at complaints as they relate to age gives a new perspective on treating the whole person."   **Townsend Letter for Doctors**

Homeopathic Medicine for Women
An Alternative Approach to Gynecological Health Care
Trevor Smith, M.D.
ISBN 0-89281-236-2
$9.95 paperback

This guidebook brings together information and advice about homeopathic treatment of a full range of gynecological disorders. Dr. Smith provides a clear description of each disorder, including its causes and symptoms. He discusses the conventional treatment and provides a list of homeopathic remedies, indicating exactly how each remedy is to be applied for specific physical and psychological symptoms. Most importantly, he shows how women can use homeopathy as an important primary treatment in caring for their own health.

Homeopathy and Your Child
A Parent's Guide to Homeopathic Treatment from Infancy Through Adolescence
Lyle W. Morgan II, Ph.D., H.M.D.
ISBN 0-89281-330-X
$9.95 paperback

Here Dr. Morgan presents safe and effective alternatives for the treatment of the most common childhood disorders, including colic, fever, diarrhea, whooping cough, measles, and mumps, discussing a wide range of homeopathic remedies as well as controversial medical practices of immunization and antibiotic treatment.

HOMEOPATHY: FROM ALCHEMY TO MEDICINE
Elizabeth Danciger
ISBN 0-89281-290-7
$5.95 paperback

This fascinating history is the first book to search for the medieval roots of modern homeopathic medicine. In a broad view of major trends in medicine from the Renaissance through the eighteenth century, the author traces ideas that influenced Hahnemann's theory of homeopathy, focusing on the work of Paracelsus, the great sixteenth century physician and alchemist, as well as that of Van Helmon, Bacon, Newton, and other original thinkers in the field of medicine.

"...very interesting to trace, along with the author, the important thinkers and scientists whose work has contributed so much to the remarkable successes of homeopathy in the 20th century."

Health World

HOMEOPATHIC TREATMENT OF SPORTS INJURIES

Lyle W. Morgan II, Ph.D., H.M.D.

ISBN 0-89281-227-3

$8.95 paperback

Homeopathic preparations provide a fast-acting, non-invasive treatment which enables an injured athlete to quickly return to optimum performance without the disadvantage of side effects. Here, Dr. Lyle Morgan, a member of the American College of Athletic and Sports Medicine, shows how homeopathy can be an effective first line of treatment for common athletic complaints, from heat stress to swimmer's ear; from skin irritations to sprains. Referenced, indexed, and with an appendix of suppliers and related medical associations, this useful handbook is particularly valuable to coaches, trainers, parents, and athletes of every level.

"This book should do much to awaken interest in homeopathy's benefits among professionals and amateurs alike." **Bestways**

HOMEOPATHIC MEDICINE
FIRST AID AND EMERGENCY CARE

Lyle W. Morgan, Ph.D.

ISBN 0-89281-249-4

$10.95 paperback

Homeopathic remedies are ideally suited to first-aid care because of the speed with which they work (conditions often improve within minutes) and because they are entirely non-invasive and without side effects. In this book, Dr. Morgan demonstrates effective homeopathic treatment for a variety of situations in the home, school, office, or campground.

Chapters on first-aid and family care cover insect bites and stings, inflammations of the eye and ear, boils, nausea, and a host of other specific ailments. Because no two situations are exactly alike, he suggests more than one treatment for any given condition, and provides illustrative case histories to help you determine which approach will achieve the best and quickest results.

Dr. Morgan addresses a wide range of the most common health emergencies, including shock, fractures, dislocations, and soft-tissue injuries. Anyone with a foundation in first-aid training can follow his basic guidelines and offer timely homeopathic treatment to best effect.

Handbook of Homeopathy

Gerhard Koehler
ISBN 0-89281-345-8
$12.95 paperback

Based on lectures given by the author, a homeopathic physician for twenty years, to medical students at Freiburg University in Germany, this book is directed to practitioners, but holds a wealth of information for anyone interested in learning more about the science of homeopathy.

Beginning with the position of homeopathy within the overall practice of medicine, Koehler explains the principles of homeopathy as set forth by Samuel Hahnemann, the methods of producing homeopathic remedies, diagnosis, and observation, including a variety of case studies.

Koehler also includes commentary on Hahnemann's *Chronic Diseases* and *Organon of Practical Medicine*. An extensive bibliography of the most important works in English, German, and French makes *Handbook of Homeopathy* an excellent resource for further study.

These and other Inner Traditions/Healing Arts Press titles are available at many fine bookstores or, to order directly from the publisher, send a check or money order for the total amount, payable to Inner Traditions, plus $2.50 shipping and handling for the first book and $1.00 for each additional book to:

Inner Traditions
P.O. Box 388
Rochester, VT 05767